HELP YOUR DOCTOR HELP YOU

WALTER C. ALVAREZ, M.D.

Cover Photograph
From HEALERS OF OUR AGE Portfolio
Copyright Karsh, Ottawa

CELESTIAL ARTS
Millbrae, California

CELESTIAL ARTS
231 Adrian Road
Millbrae, California 94030

First Printing, July 1976
Made in the United States of America

Library of Congress Cataloging in Publication Data

Alvarez, Walter Clement, 1884
Help your doctor help you.

1. Physician and patient. 2. Medical care
1. Title [DNLM: 1. Medicine–Popular works.
WB120A471h]
R727.3.A48 610.69'6 76-11342
ISBN 0-89087-169-8

1 2 3 4 5 6 — 81 80 79 78 77 76

CONTENTS

Why I Have Written This Book

During my seventy years of experience with sick people I have often been distressed to learn that many thousands of these patients had traveled from doctor to doctor and spent countless dollars seeking help while getting little or no relief. How can this be possible? Because, with little knowledge of the structure of the body and a lack of understanding of medical terms, they had told the story of their illness with so few details and such lack of accuracy that the doctor could not guess what was wrong with them. As a result, often his diagnosis and his treatment was for the wrong disease and therefore did no good and may, in fact, even have done harm.

How a stomach specialist became a diagnostician and occasional psychiatrist.

In 1926, when I started to work at the Mayo Clinic in Rochester, Minnesota, I was made a Senior Consultant in the first gastroenterology (stomach/intestinal disorders) section because I had done research in that field of medicine for thirteen years. But by 1940 I found myself working more and more often as a diagnostician and frequently, as a psychiatrist.

The reason this happened is because people who suffer from nervous abdominal aches and pains or abdominal bloating and soreness *assume* they must have stomach trouble, and so come to the *stomach section.* Actually some three thousand of the patients I saw were suffering from migraine, which also can cause nausea and vomiting. Also, a high percentage of the people with indigestion who came to me had a form of nervous indigestion and needed psychiatric help.

Along the way, another thing happened that changed my professional life. A considerable number of the nervous patients who came to the Clinic, after a thorough study, were told that there was nothing the matter with them, and many, hating to go home without any help, asked, "Isn't there some kind-hearted man around here who would be willing to struggle again with our problems and try to find some way to help us?" As the years passed, more and more often my associates would say, "Yes, Dr. Alvarez likes to struggle with problems, and often he finds out what to do about them." And so those patients were turned over to me.

Mayo Clinic has a wonderful reputation for curing people and as a result many people come from all over the world to the Clinic. They bring with them some of the most confounding problems imaginable. It always concerned me greatly when all the lab tests were taken, and the examinations were made, if "nothing" was found to be causing the problem. I could never say "There is nothing the matter with you." Instead, I explained that the reports of all the tests had been normal, indicating that none of the organs of the body were diseased. Sometimes, we were unable to help a patient. Quite often in such cases, however, months and even years later I would learn the real cause of the problem and usually it involved something the patient had not revealed to us.

One shortcut to a quick and surprisingly accurate diagnosis

I will always be grateful to my dear friend, Dr. Charlie Mayo who, early in my career gave me a bit of advice that has served me in good stead and helped me to make hundreds of diagnoses very easily or at least gave me a clue which I had only to follow-up with examination or tests. He said, "Al, when you can't tell what is causing a man's spells of illness, ask his wife. Half the time she'll tell you in short order." That is so true.

Not long after, in came a rancher who complained of spells of nausea and vomiting, the cause of which had not been found by able doctors who had examined him. I was equally baffled, for we had put him through every conceivable test at the Mayo Clinic and we too found nothing wrong.

Then I remembered Dr. Charlie's advice which at the time I had only chuckled over. I took the man's wife aside and asked, "What do you suppose these spells are due to?" And angrily she said, "I don't know what that darn fool hopes to accomplish, wasting our time and money. He knows darn well what causes those spells. He goes on binges of chewing tobacco and swallowing the juice and it makes him sick every time!"

That certainly sounded like a logical explanation to me so I asked the man if it was true. He said, "Yes, I guess so." Then sadly he added, "But I had so hoped you'd find some other cause so I could go on chewing."

Often a physician can help even if he cannot cure

A physician can cure sometimes, often he can relieve pain and almost always he can give comfort and hope. Many of my most grateful patients I was not able to cure completely, but I was able to help the person by teaching him/her to live more comfortably with some chronic or recurrent disease like an arthritis, or a migraine or a gout.

Providing health information

In my own practice I found myself repeating over and over the same general facts and advice to help each patient adjust and to live more comfortably with a chronic illness or with a temporary disability. From experience I learned the more a patient knows about his own body, its functions and malfunctions, the better off he is. But repeatedly I heard patients who came to the Mayo Clinic from tremendously capable doctors in their hometowns say, "Oh, if only my doctor had suggested that. . ." or "If only I had known that before." And I knew that, like me, their doctors had found it virtually impossible to tell each patient verbally all about his/her illness. Yet the patient needs to know the history, various methods of treatment and as many of the details of his ailment as is possible.

That was why, in 1951 I began to write a series of little booklets setting down as much information as I, a physician, could offer to people suffering from migraines, ulcers, arthritis, epilepsy, diabetes and many more. This came about because I had begun to write one of the first syndicated medical columns to appear in daily newspapers and readers would write in asking me to tell them more about a particular disease. As a result I became one of the first medical doctors to write for the general public. Thousands have told me they received one of the little booklets and that it helped them to cope with their particular problem, and to thank me for it.

Many advances have been made since then to provide medical information to those who need and want it. Many organizations founded for research and study of a specific disease have programs for disseminating public information concerning it also.

Another recent and innovative program is called Tel-Med which is available as a public service through various medical organizations in many areas. Tape recordings covering hundreds of subjects from birth control, croup, ulcers, anemia, heart disease, and the various forms of cancer are available. One need only dial the telephone number and ask to hear a certain tape. Since the use of the tapes is usually controlled by the county medical society in each area, they can probably provide information concerning it, including the telephone number to call.

This is just one of the many ongoing programs to make medical information available and it is a good indication that people are seeking information and are interested in obtaining better knowledge to live healthier, more meaningful lives.

Chapter One

Needless Suffering and Expense

Years ago I saw an attractive woman of thirty-five who had spent nearly three months in a hospital. She suffered greatly from spells of painful abdominal bloating. Twice these spells got so bad, and she became so ill, that our normally conservative surgeons decided they must explore her abdomen to save her from death by peritonitis. But they found no diseased organ.

I came by to see her often and made friends with this woman because I sensed something was very wrong. Her husband never showed up and she would never tell me anything about him, nor would she tell of any early illnesses in her life. Several times I pleaded with her to tell me if there had been a tragedy in her life but always she assured me there had been none, and there was none now. Repeatedly she denied that she knew of any problem which might be a cause for her illness. Finally, she got well enough to return home, hundreds of miles away, but I felt we had never discovered the true source of her problem.

Much to my surprise, a few months later she returned,

obviously in fine health. She said she had come to apologize to me and to clear her conscience for having failed to confide in me. She had almost forgotten the severe migraines of her teen-age years which had left her when she reached her twenties. They had returned when her husband began having spells of mild insanity. Her husband's behavior frightened her but she had attributed the return of the migraines to her fear of her husband and therefore had not told us about it; she had told us only of abdominal pain. Shortly after she had returned home her husband died and by the time his affairs were settled and she had recovered from the shock of his death, both the migraines and the abdominal bloating had disappeared. If only she had told me and our surgeons about the migraines and the crazy husband we could have saved her two operations, thousands of dollars and a great deal of suffering.

It is not uncommon for such symptoms to occur in patients with a history of previous migraines, and to be brought on again by a new but continuing stressful situation.

For example, another attractive, married but childless, active business woman had much the same alarming spells of abdominal pain. So intense were her attacks that each were suggestive of an acute appendicitis. Neither tests nor thorough examinations revealed the cause for the abdominal pain. Every day for a week I kept asking her of past discomforts or illnesses and if she had any idea what had triggered her present trouble. Finally, I got the same story of early migraines as the previous patient had revealed. In this case however, I learned the woman's mother, who was very dear to her, was slowly dying of cancer. She spent a lot of time caring for her and felt so frustrated and sad it brought back the severe migraines. I gave her the medication for migraine and in a few days she went home, the headaches greatly relieved and the abdominal pains gone.

In this case, had we not learned the facts, an unnecessary appendectomy might have been performed. Such surgery and hospitalization would only have added to the problems of this fine woman as well as deprived her mother of the comfort and love of her daughter during her final days.

Nothing is too personal to tell your doctor

People are frequently reluctant to disclose anything about venereal disease or the fact that there is insanity or epilepsy in their family. Unfortunately, these and several other diseases have a stigma attached to them.

It is imperative to trust your doctor and to give him details which may be the only way he has of properly diagnosing the problem, even when that entails revealing intimate and very personal secrets. One of the reasons venereal disease runs rampant and is so difficult to control is because people are too ashamed to tell the doctor the reason for their problems.

Many years ago I had a very fine and interesting friend, a bachelor and a college graduate, who picked up syphillis. Probably, like thousands of men caught in that situation, he, a prominent citizen, was reluctant to tell the story on himself. From his medical and family history, and from his description of his illness, nothing indicated to his doctor what the problem might be, and therefore he did not get a blood test made for that disease. Had the man said to the first doctor he went to, "I suspect I picked up some sort of venereal disease from a woman with whom I slept recently," I am pretty sure he would have lived many more years, and certainly happier years. But he did not and as a result, when he became midly psychotic, he was not treated correctly. When his mental health began to fail I could not help him because he became so violent-tempered with me that I couldn't do anything for him. After some three years of ailing, my friend became insane, and spent the last four years of his life in a mental institution.

I need hardly emphasize here how useless it is to go with a sexual problem to a doctor and then not say what the problem is. A doctor is extremely aware of human sexuality and its effects and is not going to be shocked or to feel disgust or repulsion by anything he is told. Through his education and years of experience there is little he hasn't heard. But most importantly, the doctor cannot help the patient if he is not told what has gone wrong and why it went wrong. He must know the facts.

For instance, a man once came to me in a terribly distressed state carrying a load of guilt that was affecting his health because he could neither eat nor sleep. He went to Confession regularly and told his priest of the unusual and diverse ways in which he was having sex with the woman he loved and who enjoyed and encouraged these affairs. The priest repeatedly gave him a terrible talking to, assuring him he would go to hell for his weakness and sinful behavior. When I discussed this at length with the patient and showed him books about medicine and the Bible which proved there was not a word in the Bible about what he had done, he went home a new man, no longer obsessed with guilt.

In another case a man came to me who was impotent because of premature ejaculation. After a thorough examination and extensive family history I suspected that he might be suffering from a non-convulsive epilepsy. The electroencephalograph (an electronic device which measures the activity of brain waves) proved this to be true and fortunately with the proper medicine I was able to relieve the problem. He was gloriously happy and well.

One small clue

Frequently, when I have been questioning a very nervous patient and getting nowhere, suddenly that person has inadvertently told me something, some small clue, that has soon led me to the proper diagnosis.

One day I had been struggling along, trying to find out why a very nervous business woman of thirty-four was having dizzy spells, short spells of nausea and pain in her chest radiating down her left arm. Other symptoms also suggested that nerves were playing tricks with some of her muscles here and there. She told me that several internists, psychiatrists, neurologists and ear specialists had studied her carefully but all had failed to find what was wrong.

After making no progress for perhaps half an hour, I asked her how she was getting along on her job. She seemed enthusiastic about it but remarked that she was often late to work and that was creating a problem. Upon pursuing this, since it didn't seem logical for a woman who enjoyed her work to habitually arrive late at the office, I learned she spent an inordinate amount of time washing her hands each morning and that somehow, in her mind, she associated all of this scrubbing of her hands with her fear that her father might have another heart attack. This suggested to me that she might have some psychotic background. I then learned that her father had the violent rages that afflict some epileptics, which of course may also have contributed to his heart attack. Since I believe epilepsy to be inherited, I sent the young woman down for tests and very shortly she too came back with the diagnosis of non-convulsive epilepsy. Fortunately, with medication for the control of epilepsy the patient was soon free of her affliction. Had I not found a clue in her psychotic behavior she might still be suffering with the dizzy spells, nausea and chest pains.

Remember . . .

The information *you* provide your doctor is vital to his making the proper diagnosis. It may be of tremendous importance in his interpretation of your symptoms, his decision to make certain lab tests, and even in deciding whether or not surgery is necessary. *He must know the facts.*

An illness that was cured years ago and which is now almost forgotten can be important since medical research has established patterns of recurrence or later complications. *Your telling him* will probably be the only clue your doctor may have to lead him to a correct diagnosis.

Be assured, any reputable physician will neither betray your confidence nor will he express any judgment of or lack of respect for you because of what you reveal to him. Most likely you will have gained the help and professional knowledge of someone with whom you can freely discuss your concerns.

If your doctor does not seem concerned about a detail which you had thought was important, he is probably satisfied that it is not relevant to your illness. However, should he pursue a small clue which does not seem important to you, tell him everything you can and answer his specific questions as accurately as possible. His years of training and experience have provided him with knowledge that may be the key to proper diagnosis and treatment.

Chapter Two

The Importance of an Accurate Family History

My advice to persons who are about to go to a doctor is to be prepared to provide him with the facts and then let the doctor decide what the problem is. After all, he has probably spent nine years learning to do that, in addition to his years of practical experience through his patients, and therefore ought to be much better at it than you are. Sometimes I have felt patients thought out their problems before their appointment and then came to me only for confirmation of their opinion. Some have even gone to great lengths to explain their reasons and defend the conclusions they have drawn.

It is imperative that one keep an objective mind and not go to a doctor with the intention of telling him what the problem is. Your physician will most likely ask you what *you think* is wrong, and by all means, you must answer that question as honestly and accurately as possible, because he will give your opinion proper consideration in his evaluation.

Particularly, if a doctor shows that what he wants from you is a good family history, do give it to him, with as many of the details as is possible.

Routine histories

As I write this I am reminded of an eminent physician who, after trying to study the frequency of the inheritance of epilepsy by using routine histories which he borrowed from hospitals, concluded that records of family history gathered as a matter of course by interns who have little interest in the particular case are of no value. It is frequently the practice in large hospitals or clinics, as part of the admittance procedure, for an intern to be assigned the task of taking a history. He asks "Have you or any member of your family had any of the following?" Then without pausing for breath he reads, "Allergy, asthma, blood disease, boils, chest pain, convulsions, cold or sore throat, cough, diabetes, epilepsy, fainting spells, flu, any infectuous disease, gall stones, hay fever, heart disease, hepatitis, high blood pressure, kidney disease, or diseases of the liver, leukemia, malaria, any malignancy, mononucleosis, stomach ulcers, tuberculosis, veneral disease or yellow jaundice," to which the patient automatically answers "No." Without further questions, the intern writes "none."

This, of course is an extreme example. In the event you are seeing a specialist or general practitioner for the first time he will most likely want to take a rather complete record. I have admired a woman gynecologist of whom I have heard, who, before even starting to take a family history or past medical record impresses upon her patient the importance of it by saying: "Now I am going to ask you some questions about your past medical history and that of your family. I am *not* doing this for the sake of *my* health, I am doing it for the sake of *your health.* It is *not* just a routine exercise but will probably have direct bearing upon what we will learn about your present condition. Now listen carefully and if either you or a member of your family has had any of these problems, stop me and tell me the circumstances in as much detail as possible. Now then: allergy?"

Understanding the necessity

Some diseases can be diagnosed from a physical examination and some can be diagnosed only with laboratory tests. More and more tests are being devised to make diagnosis easier and more accurate, but there is certain information which only the patient can provide. Remember, your doctor is only human and cannot guess what is in your mind or background.

From years of experience I have learned that a sick headache often is indicative of migraine; that a patient who drops to the floor in a convulsion usually has epilepsy; that a man with "hunger pain" frequently has a duodenal ulcer; and that a patient who falls out of a chair and for awhile is a bit woozy probably has had a little stroke. When I see a patient with one of these symptoms there is little question in my mind concerning what is most probably wrong, but I then get an x-ray or laboratory work done to confirm my suspicion and to be sure the patient hasn't something else wrong as well.

A doctor needs *all* the information to get a total picture of his patient's health or lack of it; a family and case history, a physical examination and any necessary laboratory tests. He is dependent upon you for the former. Surely you don't want to talk to him in such a way that he will treat you futilely for a disease you don't have while the real problem goes unchecked. Unfortunately hundreds of thousands of patients do exactly that. One of the reasons this can happen is because patients have not been sufficiently impressed with the importance of an accurate family history. Think about your own personal family. Do you know why your father's brother died in his early thirties? Or do you know how your mother lost her mother when she was only ten years old? You have probably heard the sad story that as a child she had no mother to care for her, but do you know how it happened? Oftentimes these painful memories are difficult to discuss with someone you love very much and for whom they will bring back sadness. But frequently there is an aunt, a cousin or some other member of the family who was not as emotionally attached who will be able to tell you very vividly how, when your mother was only ten, her mother came to the dinner table one evening and in the midst of family conversation, fell to the floor with a fatal stroke. She may also tell you your grandmother was overweight and had high blood pressure. You may learn that your uncle who died very young had been a diabetic from early infancy, and was almost totally blind.

Although these facts may seem unimportant to you as long as you and your family are enjoying good health, this information may be crucial when for example, your child's school nurse should call to say he has slumped into a coma at his desk. One of the first questions your doctor will probably want an answer to is whether or not there is incidence of diabetes in your family.

Natural reticence in confiding information

In addition to not realizing the importance of providing such facts, many patients find it difficult to tell the doctor the truth.

If one of my relatives had decided to get a divorce, for example, the chances are great that I would never have asked what went wrong, and they would not have offered to tell me. Neither do people like to tell anyone of an epileptic aunt, an insane grandfather or an alcoholic brother. We even have a name for such situations which families avoid discussing . . . they are called *family skeletons* and are *kept in the closet.*

Is epilepsy inherited?

Occasionally I read where even a professor in a university writes that epilepsy is not inherited. But this is very strange to me. Years ago when I looked through the literature I found 133 articles that mentioned this subject, and 132 said that epilepsy is inherited. Fifteen of the writers said that they found it inherited in about sixty percent of the cases.

As mentioned previously, family histories taken routinely in hospitals are not accurate enough to be considered as research. One of the reasons patients automatically respond by saying "No" without elaboration is that frequently he or she simply does not *know* the answer but does not mention *that fact* either. I am hopeful the time is coming when medical schools will teach all their students the futility of this type of questioning, since I am convinced people can be educated on the importance of providing complete and accurate information but need the encouragement and, in fact, the insistence of the medical profession concerning it.

Years of experience have proven to me that heredity is an important factor. I am not alone. Many years ago I visited Dr. O. P. Kimball in Detroit who was a doctor for a school for epileptic children. He told me that in many cases only when he got to know the parents and they became grateful to him for his kind care of their child, did he gain their complete confidence. Once this friendship and trust was established he began to piece together an honest study of the family history of the epileptic child and almost always there were relatives with epilepsy or associated symptoms.

The fact is, researchers have now found in the families of epileptics a 38% incidence of alcoholism, 35% where family members were "violent-tempered," a 32% incidence of insanity and 21% mentally retarded or "not quite right."

Relatives of the psychotic

I had not been practicing medicine very long before I began to recognize a type of patient who, while not disturbed enough mentally to go into a mental hospital even for a short time was so erratic and difficult in his or her behavior at times as to seem a bit psychotic.

Soon I was working hard, learning all I could about the ancestry of such people, and generally I found disturbed relatives. Unfortunately, many of the people who refuse to believe in the inheritance of a bad nervous system seem to have failed to notice that a fine type of brain can also be inherited. I feel that much of the success that comes to a family is attributable to a good mental inheritance and the ability and tendency of everyone to keep busy with worthwhile work.

Inherited does not mean incurable

Many people, upon hearing the word "inherited" or "hereditary disease" automatically throw up their hands and think, "Well, that's that! Nothing to be done about it." This is a total misconception. In the first place, it is important to emphasize that usually it is not a disease itself that is inherited but a *tendency* toward a disease. Hundreds of thousands of people inherit a *tendency to diabetes.* If, over a period of many years, such a susceptible person becomes very fat from overeating and puts great strain on his insulin-forming cells, it is quite likely that he will get diabetes. However, if his doctor knows of this tendency within the family and cautions him to eat moderately and to watch his weight so that it does not get out of hand, he may live a perfectly normal and active life and never get diabetes.

Similarly, a person who is aware that there is a tendency to psychoses within the family, if he practices good mental hygiene and particularly if he has a capable physician who knows his situation and to whom he can go for guidance, may live a long, normal and satisfying life.

One must not assume that because a disease is hereditary in nature it is untreatable or hopeless. Some definitely inherited diseases, such as diabetes and pernicious anemia can now be kept under control for a lifetime.

Unfortunately, because of the misinterpretation of the words "hereditary disease," many doctors are hesitant to mention it. Naturally it is easier to help an essentially normal person who through strain, grief, insomnia or overwork has developed a neurosis than it is to help a patient who has always been ill-tempered, eccentric, and possibly difficult and undisciplined. But both doctor and patient must be aware of the encouraging fact that many of these tendencies toward hereditary problems can be treated and overcome.

Professional confidence

Another reason a few people may be reticent about confiding in their doctor is that they may be afraid the doctor might tell someone what they disclose to him in private. This is extremely unlikely.

For more than sixty-five years I have been writing about patients and giving speeches in which I frequently use case histories to offer an example or to stress a point. Only once have I gotten into trouble for doing that and then I got a royal tongue-lashing from a member of my own family, although the situation I described was more amusing than embarrassing. Apparently a doctor who was a very close friend of our family and knew us all very well, guessed about whom I was talking and teased her about it. This wouldn't be likely to happen in any normal doctor-patient relationship because doctors are constantly aware of the need for professional confidence.

It is customary when a doctor publishes a picture of a patient in a medical journal that the patient's face is covered or blocked out. When a patient's case history is used as an example in an article or a book, always the names and some of the non-essential facts are changed so the person cannot be recognized. This is standard procedure throughout the medical profession.

So once we understand the *need* for a family medical history and rid ourselves of the inhibitions of *dragging the family skeletons out of the closet* when necessary, we must set about *obtaining* a family history.

Compiling the family history

Today many families are scattered throughout the country because of the extremely mobile society in which we live and this certainly makes it more difficult and in some cases impossible to gather all the facts. But it is important and everyone should make an effort to obtain as much accurate information as possible.

From your own memory and knowledge you can jot down the things that have happened in your own lifetime in your immediate family. When you go to visit distant relatives, or are going to be in the vicinity where they live, make it a point to call on them and renew your acquaintance. If you have only heard your family speak of them, introduce yourself and become acquainted. Don't hesitate to explain why you want medical information about your relatives; they will understand. Assure them of your confidence, and ask what they can tell you. You may be surprised by what you learn, and it may provide great insight into present or future health problems.

Be sure to *write down* the facts as soon as possible; don't depend on your memory. Most parents have had the experience of keeping a record of a child's vaccinations and inoculations; one learns not to try to keep a "mental note" of it, particularly if there are several children in the family. What with DPT shots, smallpox, measles, polio, flu shots and, of course, the boosters, one soon realizes the wisest course of action is to make a permanent written record. In many areas some booster shots are given through public school health departments which further increases the need for accurate home records. Then the next time Junior steps on a rusty nail and the doctor asks, "When did he last have a tetanus shot?" you can give him an exact answer rather than trying to remember if last fall was when Junior got the tetanus or if that was when Rover got the rabies shot. A *written* record of family medical history is similarly important.

The task of setting down a family medical history will be made easier if some member of the family has worked out a family tree or family history, as has become very popular recently. Then it becomes a matter of making inquiry within the family of the details of illnesses and deaths of the family members. Taking the time and making the effort to compile this record will be well worth the trouble. You will have occasion to refer to it often as you grow older and it may be an invaluable record to pass on to your children for their health and for their children's health.

Remember . . .

Go to your doctor with an open mind ready to provide the information he requests. *Do not* diagnose your own case and then give him only the information that supports your opinion. There may be a vital bit of information which he will recognize that you may have either overlooked or of which you have not understood the significance.

An accurate and complete knowledge of family illness or disease is important and you should not be embarrassed or reluctant to discuss any personal or family member's condition with your physician. Nor should there be any concern that a competent and respected physician might repeat anything that is told to him as a professional confidence.

The fact that there is an inherited *tendency* toward a dread disease *does not mean* it is incurable or cannot be successfully controlled.

We must recognize the need for a complete medical history and then set about compiling it using the sources available by talking with and asking questions of other family members.

This information should be recorded and kept in a safe place just as you would keep any other records which are important to the health and welfare of your family. Over the years this record should be brought up-to-date to reflect recent developments and it should be passed on as children leave home to establish homes and families of their own.

Chapter Three

Additional Sources of Inaccurate Information

The average person usually has scant knowledge of the body and its functions. If one were to examine his vocabulary of medical terminology and attempt to trace where he first heard and learned the words he uses, I suspect he would find an almost frightening lack of correct definition and even more alarming would be the sources from which they came.

Many of the words used to express a physical condition are learned within the family while youngsters are growing up. Almost everyone can recall instances in their childhood when they became sick to their stomach, vomited, ran a fever, possibly had diarrhea, muscular pain and generally felt *awful all over.* Mother probably said "You have the flu," and you were put to bed, kept warm and encouraged to drink a lot of broth. If you had been playing with the boy next door and he caught it, his mother may have called it the grippe. Once you felt all right again these early experiences with illness were most likely forgotten, but somewhere in your subconscious you formed vague definitions of the words that described the symptoms and illness. You may also have memories of a biology class taken years ago from which to draw, but word meanings become cloudy and less than accurate. Additionally dissolved into your vocabulary are other people's descriptions of illnesses and their often inaccurate identification of parts of their bodies and description of what happened to *them* which may or may not have any similarity to *your* particular problems. Oftentimes a person uses words that he has heard from a doctor; however his use frequently is directed toward a particular instance and may not encompass the entire definition or may not be indicative of the broad meaning of the word.

Today another frequent source of medical information is the television commercials for brand name non-prescription remedies which use intricate diagrams of violently churning stomachs and headaches illustriously depicted complete with air hammers, clanging bells and sirens creating mental disharmony and pain. Immediately, as antacids gush into the stomach or pain relievers reach the bloodstream, miracles of relief and calm take place. Sinus cavities, bronchial tubes, the inner ear and muscle spasms are likewise brought to us in living color. Although they are not necessarily medically inaccurate, liberties are taken by the advertising agencies in exposing various organs through cartoon drawings.

Additionally, a great variety of maladies, illnesses and accidents are aired through daily and weekly *entertainment* shows based on doctors' lives and practices; others depend upon a hospital, medical clinic, emergency or paramedic team as the theme for the program. Although the producers of these shows do go to great lengths to authenticate the details of the shows, the viewers are picking up words used in context without learning their complete meaning.

Naturally everyone wants to express himself as effectively as possible. But when it comes to medical terminology it is terribly important to be certain of the definition of the words you use. Generally your doctor will question you to be sure that you are understanding each other correctly, but all too often the wrong impression is given. Long ago I learned, if I felt my patient did not appear to fully understand, to explain the problem to him in very simple lay terms until I was *certain* he understood.

LOCATING THE PROBLEM

Actual location of the source of the problem in a specific area of the body can cause confusion. I have found it helpful to have a patient *show me* by pointing to the place on his body to which he was referring. Once, much to my chagrin and the total embarrassment of the professor of a medical school, this lesson was brought home vividly and before a large number of people. I had been asked to give a talk on duodenal (twelve inches of bowel just beyond the stomach) ulcer to a hundred medical school students. The professor had provided me with a patient on whom to demonstrate the ulcer.

The man was a Serbian miner with a poor knowledge of the English language and apparently there had been some misunderstanding in the case history taken previously. In front of all the medical students and their professor, I asked the gentleman to show me with his hand where the pain was; he pointed first to the right side of his back near the middle, then ran his hand down, following the course of a spinal nerve to the right side of his pelvis! Needless to say we were all quite shocked and promptly obtained and examined an x-ray film of the man's spine. At the point where he had first placed his hand was the picture of a diseased vertebra. An x-ray film of his stomach indicated a slight deformity and years before he may have had a little ulcer.

Unfortunately, in my day, medical students were not always taught to ask the patient with a pain in his *stomach* to point to where that was. I learned it for myself and I feel certain the medical students who were present that day never fail to ask that question of their patients.

His life depended upon it

I remember one man who, poor fellow, lost his life because he made a similar mistake. He had been treated for a year for "stomach trouble" largely because that's what he told his doctor he had. Like many people I have examined, he *thought* stomach meant the entire abdomen. When I asked him to show me where the pain was he pointed to his pelvis. A rectal examination revealed a cancer much too old and too scattered to be successfully removed by surgery.

A little detective work

Another case had a much happier ending. A man who led an active life and enjoyed good health came to me one day in a state of great anxiety. He had complained of a pain in his upper chest and his family doctor thought it was arising from his heart. He was naturally quite upset since if he did have heart trouble he felt that he would have to *take it easy* and he would have to change his entire way of life. When he showed me exactly where the pain was I saw it was high up toward his right shoulder. Then I felt the tissue and found that what he really had was a very sore muscle.

I said, "Let's see, today is Tuesday; what extraordinary exercise did you have with your arm over the weekend?"

"Well I spent the whole weekend painting the kitchen and the garage," he promptly answered. There, of course, was the cause of the pain in his upper chest muscle. A bit embarrassed, he laughed and said, "Now why didn't I think of that!" Naturally, his anxiety concerning his heart was immediately relieved and in just a few days the soreness was gone too.

DESCRIBING THE PROBLEM

Once the source of the problem is located, we must then find the correct words with which to describe it.

Once a wealthy pre-Castro sugar baron came to me. He had recurring episodes which were very distressing to him. He said he had diarrhea and he and his wife had been traveling around, going to almost every major medical clinic in the United States for help, but getting none.

When he came to the Mayo Clinic he was directed to our diarrhea specialist, probably the best man in his field in the entire world. As in the other clinics he had visited, the bowel was examined through a tube, an x-ray film was made, the feces were examined and his digestion was studied. All of this took two or three weeks, and there was still no clue as to what was causing the diarrhea.

He was about to be sent off without help but as a last resort I was asked to see him. He was very dejected. "For God's sake," he said, "I'm so tired and fed up. We have been traveling around and I don't want to have to go to yet another clinic. Can't you help me?"

I had thoroughly reviewed the man's history, his tests and x-rays, but could find nothing the others had missed. I decided to utilize Dr. Charlie's old plan and asked the man to wait. I got his wife and took her into a private room where we could talk. We chatted for a few minutes and then I said, "You know, your husband doesn't seem to be able to tell me exactly what brings these spells of diarrhea on or what happens. Can you tell me about it?"

"Well," she said, "I'm glad you asked me that. The other doctors always fussed around with him and he didn't want me to have anything to do with it so he always left me in the waiting room. I've been thinking about it and I'm not sure he has diarrhea at all, at least I wouldn't call it that. But for heaven's sake, don't tell him any of this. He would be furious with me."

I assured her that her husband would never know and then she said, "He gets scared. There is a lot of insanity on his side of the family. Both his father and his uncle died in a mental hospital. When he gets a spell of depression he becomes afraid that he is going to go the same way they did and he gets frantic. It scares the pants off him. He'll be sitting there, reading with me, and all of a sudden he gets one of these spells and jumps up and starts running around the house like a crazy man. Then he will rush into the bathroom to the toilet and it is like his bowel sort of explodes. Then he will be over his spell and he doesn't have a bowel movement again for four or five days."

"Well, that's not diarrhea," I said. "It takes four or five days for the bowel to fill, so if this happens when he is depressed and then he has spells of anxiety, he needs medicine for depression, not diarrhea."

"Well, that's what his spells are!" she said. "But he just can't talk about that insane family of his!" I thanked her and gave the man medication to fight off his depressions. He quit having the spells and went home happy. What a shame he couldn't describe to his other doctors what he called "diarrhea." He wouldn't have wasted six months and thousands of dollars on useless examinations and tests.

Differentiating between similar symptoms

People frequently find it difficult to tell the difference between nervous indigestion, an ulcer, and digestive disorders brought on by other problems. Quite often the patient will identify all of these as "an ulcer."

However, if a patient tells a story of indigestion, with flatulence, nausea, heartburn, a vague distress in the abdomen which comes anytime of the day or night, I may suspect he/she has what is often called nervous indigestion.

This is usually due to some acute annoyance at home or at work, possibly overwork or fatigue.

If a man tells me of spells of pain in his upper central abdomen which seem to come just before lunchtime and which go away as soon as he drinks some milk or eats however, I can be pretty sure that he really has an ulcer. Often this type of patient tells me of bitter opposition and jealousy with which he must put up at the office, or that the pain comes after a serious argument with his wife.

In either case, I know what tests to give the patient and what x-rays should be taken. Once this is done and the diagnosis is confirmed, the proper remedy can be utilized. As a part of the remedy, if I can work with the patient to find the source of the annoyance, frequently he or she can make a change will rid him or her of the problem.

In some cases the only solution is for the patient to change jobs, or even to get a divorce from a spouse that creates such intense anxiety. In one case, though, it was simply to insist that a teenager in an adjoining bedroom turn off a radio which frequently played all night—to the great distress and aggravation of the parent. However, all things must be considered. Obviously, an ulcer is one thing; it may require surgery. Nervous indigestion is quite another. There are many illnesses which produce similar symptoms and therefore are frequently confused, particularly when the patient is unable to give an adequate description of the problem.

THIRD PARTY COMMUNICATION

The pitfalls of improper communication are even greater when the patient is unable to speak for himself. Often it is a parent who must try to convey to the doctor the distress and accompanying symptoms for a child. Or a young man or woman might speak for a parent disabled by a stroke or other incapacitating illness. Here the communication problems are compounded by a lack of firsthand knowledge, the misuse of medical terminology, and insufficient knowledge of the body parts, organs and their functions.

Mislead by a child

One mother told me a story of her frustration with her five-year-old daughter who had an earache. The child was a bit precocious anyway and had a surprising vocabulary for her age. The doctor examined the little girl carefully and prescribed medication for the earache. In examining her nasal passages he remarked to the mother, "I think she has probably had a little congestion too."

Not realizing that the little girl had promptly picked up a new word, the mother replied, "Oh, I don't think so; I certainly would have noticed that." About that time the little blonde turned wide-eyed to her mother and said, "I've had a lot of congestion." Surprised, the mother questioned her further but she emphatically nodded her head and told both the doctor and the mother that she definitely, and frequently, had congestion.

The doctor wrote out another prescription, this one for the relief of congestion, and soon mother and daughter were on their way, stopping at the drug store to have the prescriptions filled.

That evening at the dinner table the mother was chagrined to hear the little girl, wide-eyed and wondering, ask her father, "Daddy, what's *congestion*?"

There are a tremendous number of childhood problems which can easily become confused. For example, many parents have been frightened into rushing a child to the doctor, thinking it was having an attack of acute appendicitis, only to learn later that without their knowledge the child had consumed great amounts of a variety of "goodies" which were causing the conflict in the child's tummy.

When our daughter had acute appendicitis, I took her to the hospital at three o'clock at night and she was operated on by six since the storm was so acute there was no question. However I asked an eminent children's specialist how he determined the difference between the stomachache of a child who had eaten too much of some indigestible food and the one who had acute appendicitis. I'll never forget his statement that the stomachache will probably go away by midnight while an acute appendicitis will keep the child and his mother awake all night. Of course, if there is any question in a parent's mind that it might be appendicitis, it is wise to get the early opinion of their doctor.

Incapacitated elderly

When an incapacitated adult's symptoms and suffering must be described by a third party, the circumstances can be very sad. I remember a woman who was brought to me by her fine young son who told me she had been treated for a supposed ulcer in her stomach. The treatment did not help her.

Although she was not an old woman she did not offer any information herself but allowed her son to do all the talking for her. Her face seemed haggard and dull. I asked her a few questions which she answered so poorly that it was obvious her brain had been damaged somewhat. When I asked her to show me with her hand where she felt pain, she pointed to her left hip! Because pain in the stomach never comes in that area I knew that her trouble was not an ulcer in the stomach. Probably she pointed to her hip because in her deadened state of mind she had bumped it.

I asked the young man to tell me what had happened, if this change in his mother had come on recently. He said "Yes, one day while mother was crossing an avenue in the city she suddenly stopped in the middle of the street and stood there until a policeman went out and brought her over to the sidewalk. She was unable to answer his questions concerning her identity so he looked in her purse, found my address and called me. I went and took her home and ever since that time she has been almost totally dependent on others."

There was little question but that the woman had suffered a little stroke while crossing the street. What was sad was that her doctor did not get that story from her son. He had depended upon an x-ray report which showed some distortion of the stomach. It is quite possible she may have had a little ulcer years before.

Many people feel that by simply delivering the physical person to a physician they have done everything they can do, but that is incorrect. The treatment that patient receives, and the amount of good that comes from it, may be greatly increased by the "homework" done in advance of the examination. When you are in the position of having to speak for an older person or for a young child it is wise to sort out all of the facts, as you know them, in advance. It would be wise to write them down, and to attempt to set down the date when the symptoms first occurred. You will probably find it easier to communicate with the older person or the child at home, to draw from them answers to questions that will most likely come up during the examination.

Giving specific information about symptoms is important in any case, but it is of particular consideration when it comes to children. For example, so many mothers have told me, either by phone or during an office call, "She had a high fever during the night."

How high was the child's temperature? Exactly what did it register on the thermometer? Often, the parent does not know, only having felt the child's forehead and determining that the child had a fever because by comparison it was warmer than her own forehead. An essential item of any family medicine cabinet should be an accurate thermometer; more importantly, it should be used and the exact degree of temperature noted. There are so many illnesses, particularly in childhood, which manifest themselves by symptoms which include running a temperature. Considered with the child's age, the degree of temperature can be serious and in fact, if the fever goes too high the child may go into convulsions.

When a person, young or old, is sick the temperature should be taken regularly, so that any change may be noted. Unless checked by a thermometer, a low grade fever may go unnoticed for a long time.

The doctor may also want to know, by way of general information, what, how often and how much the patient has eaten, so notice should be taken of how much food is offered and how much is actually consumed. Likewise, he may have questions regarding bladder elimination and bowel movements.

Whether you are yourself going to a doctor for a personal problem or are taking someone else for whom you are responsible, you should give some thought to the conversation you will have with the doctor. Think of the words you will use to describe symptoms and their location. Even checking those words in any standard household dictionary for common usage will be helpful, although such definitions will be brief.

There are many fine books, medical dictionaries and medical encyclopedias available which many people find helpful to own as part of their family library. A few of the most popular volumes which are easily understood by non-medical people are *Black's Medical Dictionary,* by William A. R. Thomson, M.D. published by Harper and Row, 1974; *The Cyclopedic Medical Dictionary,* by Clarence W. Tabor, published by Davis Co., 1973; *Dorland's Illustrated Medical Dictionary, W. B. Saunders, 1974; The Penguin Medical Encyclopedia* by Peter Wingate, 1972; and *Stedman's Medical Dictionary* published by the Williams and Wilkins Company, 1972. These and others like them contain short, simple definitions of medical terminology which you will find of great value in intelligently discussing problems with your physician.

Remember . . .

When consulting a physician, unless you are positive of the meaning of a medical term, use simple, every day language; language which both you and the doctor will interpret the same way.

Point to your body to show him *exactly* where you mean, in addition to verbally explaining the problem.

Consider unusual activities or occurrences that might have had an effect on the circumstances of your illness.

Obtain, either through a local library or buy yourself, a dictionary or an encyclopedia of medical terms. Look up the definitions of words you will use in talking with your doctor . . . even if they are words you have used all your life.

Use very great care when you are responsible for describing the illness of someone too young or otherwise unable to speak for themselves. Do your "homework" by learning as much as possible about that person's problems before you arrive at the doctor's office.

Write down all the facts which you think may be important, particularly the temperature in degrees, the time taken and the duration of the fever as well as information concerning the intake of food and liquids, and elimination.

Chapter Four

The Effect of Emotion on the Body

When people wonder about the effect of emotion on various parts of the body such as the heart, stomach and bowel, and ask if emotion can do much harm, I remind them that emotion can even kill a person.

All of which makes me hopeful that some day in college, or perhaps even in high school, young people will get lectures on the ease with which disturbed emotions can cause a severe and even fatal illness. We have all heard the expression that someone "died of a broken heart." This is more than just an old cliché. There is no doubt that disease and death can be brought about by emotional stress.

MIND OVER MATTER

When patients would not tell me about the traumatic experience that ushered in their illness, I often told them a story, a case history perhaps, to show them how severely strong emotion can interfere with the functions of various body organs. Frequently, that would help them to divulge their own problems and then together we could look for the answers.

The spell of the kahuna

One story which I have recounted frequently happened when I was very young. It taught me how the power of the mind can control the body. When I was a boy in Hawaii, my father, who was a doctor, was often upset when he could not save a kanaka (native Hawaiian) who had been told he was being "prayed to death" by a kahuna (witch doctor). At that time in the Islands if you wanted to get rid of someone you just went to a kahuna and paid him some money and he would send a message to your enemy that he was being "prayed to death." The poor fellow, because he had been raised to believe there was nothing he could do, without exception simply sat down on a mat and within ten days was dead.

Once I was standing with my father in the yard outside our house when a black man, whom I think was a Portuguese from Angola, came by. He had married the daughter of a chief and through her had acquired a ranch where he raised many cattle. He was annoyed because there were two thieves stealing his cattle. Whenever those two thieves wanted to give a big luau, or feast, they'd steal, and slaughter, more of his stock. The thieves were very popular with their friends, of course, but they never paid him a nickle for the cattle. What really aggravated him was that his cowboys knew these guys, knew what they were doing, and even attended the luaus. Twice he had the two thieves arrested but because his own cowboys refused to testify against them there were no witnesses to support the charges. His wife, the Hawaiian chieftan's daughter, had explained this to him. "Don't you know what's the matter?" she asked. "The thieves sent a message to the cowboys that if they testified they would be prayed to death by a kahuna, so you see, they are too scared to testify."

Upon hearing this my father said, "Well, if I were in your place I would make the kahuna a better offer and have *the thieves* prayed to death."

"Good idea!" the man exclaimed. He jumped on his horse and rode off.

About ten days later he came back and said to my father, "Hey, Doctor, those two thieves are dead, and it only cost me a cow and two pigs!"

But you know, my father tried his darndest to talk the natives out of that belief. He told them that the American doctors were much wiser and had much better medicine and so forth. But they would say, "No, you're a malihini (a foreigner) and you can't do anything here. I will have to die," and so they would go ahead and die. Things have changed now but it was a good example of what the mind can do!

Fear

I learned about the power of fear personally once during an epidemic of severe and often fatal influenza that raged through California. One day my wife telephoned to say that my much loved little daughter had just gone to bed with a high fever and already was so ill that she did not recognize her mother. I immediately left my office, hurried home, and took the child to the University Hospital.

Knowing that the chances were great that she would be dead in a few days, and having no drug that would cure her, I was so distressed that I could not eat. I could not sleep that night and I was physically ill for three days until my little girl started to get well. My own violent reaction to the strain convinced me of the power of my mind over my body.

Also early in my medical life I was impressed with the fact that if a person was to be operated on and said that he/she was going to die, perhaps with the first whiff of the anesthetic, he/she commonly did die in just that way.

You couldn't pay me...

When I was practicing in Northern Mexico, a wealthy middle-aged widow came into my office one day. She was in a very nervous state, trembling with anxiety and fear. She had an inn on the edge of the city, used mainly by drivers who at night left their horses and wagons in a corral next to the inn.

When, as so commonly happens with very nervous and fear-ridden patients, she would not tell me a word about what she was so afraid of, I went to her inn, and into her private apartment. There I finally got her to confess that, needing help in the running of the corral, she had married an American cowboy. Soon she discovered that he was lazy and had married her only for her money. Accordingly he wasn't much help in running the place.

Naturally, they were soon quarreling and when she found a big knife under his pillow, next to hers, she became terrified. She was sure he was planning to murder her.

I went out and chatted with the husband. As an experiment, I said, "You know, if I were in your place, you couldn't pay me to sleep on that pillow of yours. I would be scared that any night now she would get two or three of her devoted corral workers to charge in and cut my throat from ear to ear."

And he said, "You're right, I am scared." With that he jumped on a horse and soon was racing for the American border and Arizona. When I went back to tell her that he was gone, she was like a different person and got perfectly well! Which shows that sometimes a doctor can cure without giving medicine.

Anger

I recall a very dear friend whom I had known for thirty years. He was a very pleasant man who was very wealthy. But one day he came to my office and I saw that he had changed. His face was contorted; he was angry and upset. I said, "What in the world is wrong? What has hit you so hard?"

He had only two children, both of whom he loved very dearly and recently he had lost his wife. He said, "My daughter is sueing me for part of her mother's estate. I don't see why . . . I'm going to leave it to her when I die!"

I told him, "Look, you must forgive your daughter. . . do whatever is necessary to work things out with her, or this thing is going to kill you." I was certain of that and I pleaded with him and said, "For God's sake, let it go. . . give it to her and forgive her."

"No, I just can't," he said. "The way I'm made I just cannot believe a daughter ought to sue her father for her mother's estate. It makes me so mad that I can't sleep at night."

The man was so upset that first his heart went bad and then his kidneys gave out. He stayed angry, and of course he was still suffering from the loss of his wife. It was only a few weeks until he died.

A very sensitive storekeeper, a patient of mine, when sued by an angry customer, got such severe abdominal pain, bloating, heartburn and insomnia that his doctor wanted to operate; he was certain the man had an ulcer. But when the case was settled, the man was well.

Shock

One day I saw a man and his wife who had come a thousand miles, hoping desperately that I could find a cure for the cancer which he had in both lungs. I told them I would call our two best experts, but that I had little hope that a cure could be effected since the cancer was wide spread in both lungs. Within a half hour the wife dropped dead. The shock of the bad prognosis distressed her so much that she died.

Another woman, while driving her car, had an accident in which her sister whom she cared for deeply was killed. The woman felt so guilty and so terribly unhappy that she promptly committed suicide.

Trauma

Many patients do not tell their doctor that they developed their illness the day after they suffered some tragedy that upset them greatly, like a big row with someone they care for very much and who is important in their life.

Thousands of women patients were too reluctant to tell me that their illness came the day after they had had bitter arguments with their husbands. Many failed to tell me their misery came when they could not make up their minds whether or not to get a divorce. One young woman eventually told me she had fallen ill when the young man whom she was planning to marry found someone he liked better.

Month after month I have marvelled that a person whose illness followed immediately on a tragedy in their life could not have seen that it was the cause of the trouble, and that there was not much sense in going to a doctor except to get a drug to soothe them and to help them to sleep. A woman whose illness was due to the death of her adored little daughter could get well only by learning to accept the loss philosophically and to live normally again.

Faith and hope

Emotion fortunately works both ways. It can, as we have shown here, kill people but by the same token, there are many cases in which the mind, stimulated and made very hopeful by great religious faith will work a cure. This becomes very evident when a patient who is paralyzed or otherwise very ill is cured by a religious healer. The power of the mind when greatly fortified with trust and confidence can make one well.

Relief through assurance

Sometimes I have been impressed with the fact that a patient who was told that his/her thorough examination had shown no organic disease, immediately left, so satisfied and happy that he/she did not ask either for advice or medication. I recall a big husky farmer who had a chronic ache in his left groin which, although not very painful, concerned him since he was afraid it might be an indication of a serious disease. After a thorough examination I asked him what he would do if I were to assure him that he had no cancer or anything that would ever "turn into something." He reached for his coat and laughingly said, "I'd say to hell with it!" and off he went, happy.

Weir Mitchell's rest cure

For some five years, I had as a great teacher Dr. Emile Schmoll, a brilliant man who had been well-trained in some of the greatest medical centers of Europe.

When he treated a patient who was suffering greatly from nervousness, indigestion, insomnia, great anxiety, or perhaps emaciation, he used the great Dr. Weir Mitchell's Rest Cure in a sanatorium when the patient could afford it. There, for two or three weeks, the patient lay in a bed and received excellent food and excellent nursing care. The insomina was overcome with drugs and everyone about him/her was encouraging.

I remember that all but four of the many women I saw so treated were helped, and some were helped greatly. The four who were not helped all had severe sexual problems. Curiously, I can even remember the problems of two of those women. One was the wife of a business man who had begun to come home late. When she discovered that he was having an "affair" with his secretary, she went completely to pieces. My chief put her in the hospital, but three weeks later she was no better. The nurse told me, "I expect every day to find she has committed suicide."

Then I tried a desperate experiment. I asked her husband if he would mind strangling her to death. Astonished, he asked me "Why do you suggest such a thing?" I said, "Because it would be much kinder than the death you are dealing out to her now."

He thought a bit and then said, "Yes, I guess you are right. I will break it off with my secretary tomorrow." He did and started to give his wife the affection and attention that she needed for living and soon she was well.

The other woman who did not improve under this treatment puzzled my chief since she would not admit that she had any worries. However, the nurse when questioned said, "She can't get well under these circumstances. Her parents come very evening and visit her until nine. Then they go home, and a handsome young man comes and remains until we put him out at ten. Your patient is crazy about him and wants to marry him. He wants to marry her, but their parents have different religions, and won't let them get married." When I told her parents that they were the cause of her suffering, they consented to the marriage and the girl got well.

I keep pointing out that some cures which cannot be worked with medicine can be worked by helping the patient change his circumstances or by adjusting to and accepting them.

Don't lose your temper

Osler, America's greatest doctor in his day, warned people

not to lose their tempers; it not only wastes energy, it interferes with success in business, and it can ruin a person's health as well.

I have seen patients whose severe illness was brought on by their tendency to go into rages. One of the most remarkable cases of this was that of a factory foreman who came to me complaining of spells of jaundice. He eventually told me that every one of those spells had come when he had violently lost his temper with a workman.

I saw another man when he was having "spells of fever." His local doctor thought he had brucellosis, a disease of cattle, but at the Mayo Clinic that was ruled out by blood tests.

I asked his wife what she thought, and she said all his spells had followed attacks of rage. I convinced him this was damaging his health and suggested other ways of channelling his energy when he was about to become angry. Soon he was well and his relationships in business improved so much that he received a fine promotion.

Once I had as a patient a millionaire who had a tendency to go into towering rages. This would cause his blood pressure to rise and one time he became frightened that he was going to die and came to me for an examination. When I learned of his tendency to become totally infuriated I talked him into promising to do something else when he was about to lose his temper. His secretary told me later that he kept that promise with such success that it greatly increased his health and his happiness. In fact, his wife, who had been planning to divorce him, changed her mind.

When I was nineteen I had an experience which taught me this lesson personally. I caught an older man trying to steal my beloved horse and I became so angry I was tempted to jump him and break his neck. I would probably have succeeded too, since at the time I had taken up wrestling as a hobby. Fortunately, I kept myself under control and thus avoided possible serious trouble with the law. But that one burst of anger left me so exhausted for a day that I promised myself I would never lose my temper like that again but would instead keep my energies intact for useful work.

If more people knew how much bodily distress anxiety and sorrow or nervous shock can produce, they would be less likely to agree to surgery on some abdominal organ which frequently is not the source of their problem. They should look first for some other cause and when the illness comes after a great emotional storm should simply tell their doctor, "I developed this illness the day my husband told me of an affair he was having," or, "I became sick the day my father, whom I idolize, had a bad stroke" or "The day when I flunked out of college." Imagine a man who on coming in might say, "This started the day I learned my sixteen-year-old daughter was pregnant," or "The day my boy got arrested for stealing a car," or "The day my wife was diagnosed as having cancer."

Hysteria

In Mexico I cured a number of hysterically paralyzed women either with a hopeful chat, or by stimulation of the non-functioning muscles with a little faradic battery. I will never forget a woman who told me that a bolt of lightning had come through the window, striking her right foot and running up her right leg to her hip, leaving the leg paralyzed. I am sure that she was so frightened by the lightning that she became hysterical and could not get it out of her mind. I said, "We will drive it out just the same way it came in," and moved the electrode of my little battery from her right hip down to the bottom of her foot. Obviously relieved, she got up and walked.

I learned from a tense and unhappy woman how severe mental anguish can be. When I asked her how she and her mother-in-law were getting along, she went completely to pieces. She jumped up and screamed and wept hysterically. She looked as if she were going insane. This illustrates how much suffering and illness can be produced in a sensitive woman when she has to live with somone whom she greatly dislikes.

THE TRAP DISEASE

In most of these cases some sudden traumatic happening caused an immediate turn-around in the health and well-being of a person. But over the years I have watched another type of emotional circumstance with my patients. I even gave it a name, I call it the "Trap Disease." This is when personal circumstances and environment slowly involve the person over a period of time until they are caught up in a situation from which there seems no recourse and eventually they become depressed, lose their hope, and eventually their health.

I remember the first young woman who taught this to me. She was a dear little dark-eyed Irish girl from Minneapolis. She came to me with her mother who was suffering from a long terminal disease for which there was no treatment except to keep her as comfortable as possible.

The daughter cried easily, was depressed and very unhappy. She had a great depression that had been with her for some time. I could see she was losing both her emotional and physical health. In talking with her I asked "What has happened to you. When did you get so depressed."

"Well," she told me, "I've been engaged for several years and I love him very much. . .we're in love with each other and we have wanted to get married. But then my mother became ill and I have to take care of her because my father is an alcoholic. I have to stay and take care of them both. My fiancé came to me a month ago and he says we have waited long enough. He wants to get married and start a life of our own. But I can't leave them . . . I'm just *caught in a trap.*"

Some traps are different. I had a young man come to me

and his *trap disease* was financial. Fortunately this one had a happy ending! He came from Atlanta, Georgia. He complained of stomach trouble and we put him through a barrage of tests but couldn't find anything wrong with him.

After several talks he finally told me that he was badly in debt. This was in 1929, during the crash. He owed two or three thousand dollars to a man who had become very nasty and who had threatened him. The young man was actually afraid to deal with the fellow, and of course in 1929 two or three thousand dollars looked pretty big.

After I heard this I knew there wasn't much Mayo Clinic could do for him so I said, "I'm really sorry, but I am afraid the only way to cure you would be for some wealthy relative to come along and pay your debt." He agreed, and said that was most likely the cause of his problem. Several years later I had to go to Atlanta to give a speech for a hospital dedication and while I was there this fellow came up to me. He said, "Doctor, I heard you were going to be in town and I just had to come and tell you what happened. You were right. I had an uncle in Australia that we had almost forgotten. He came over for a visit and he gave me $5,000 and you know, I paid off my debt and got a new start and I haven't had any stomach trouble since."

Wasn't that marvelous?

There was another fellow who just didn't get along with his wife at all. She was a nagger and he had decided he couldn't stand her any longer and he would get a divorce. Then he met someone else and really fell in love with her. She was just what he wanted and he was eager to marry her.

But shortly before he was about to get a divorce his wife was in an automobile accident. She was in very serious condition in the hospital and it dragged on and on. He said, "I just don't feel it is right to leave her without help when she is that bad off. I'm very depressed and now I'm losing the girl I wanted to marry and that's why my health is shot!" No wonder!

One day long ago an emaciated, sad-looking young woman was brought to me by her father. I asked her what had ruined her life, and she said that a few months before she had been a healthy, happy secretary in Boston planning to be married.

Then came a letter from her "cracked on religion" mother in Chicago, saying, "Come and take care of me, I am dying." So she went, and every day since then she sat silently in a darkened room while her mother read the Bible. As if that was not enough, her boy friend wrote to say he was getting tired of waiting.

I immediately said to the father, "If you want to save your daughter's health, take her right now to the station and get her a ticket to Boston."

"All right," said the man, "that I will do," and off they went.

For years after that I got happy and very grateful letters from that girl. She said my treatment was much better than any medicine.

Seeing what a patient could not see for herself

Sometimes a person becomes so locked into their own life situation that even though they honestly try they cannot see what the problems are. This is particularly true if it is a circumstance which they think cannot be changed; they simply refuse to look in that direction.

I have had many such cases where my patient would not or could not express the emotional problem they were struggling with and on occasion, if possible, I would visit their home and then I would usually find out. Often an outsider can see the problem much more objectively.

A colleague of mine once wrote me that the wife of a very distinguished and wealthy citizen in his city had come to him with tremendous migraines. "It's really terrible," the doctor said, "and I have been unable to provide her with a particle of relief. Please be prepared for the worst; have her hospital bed ready, special nurses and so forth.'' And he added, ''I hope this case will not interfere with our friendship.''

Well, the woman came to me all right and she did indeed have migraines. She took all the relevant tests and we found nothing else wrong with her. We gave her medication to help the migraines as much as possible and I tried my darndest to figure out her problem.

''What is it in your home that sensitizes you to migraine?'' I asked because I felt certain there was some special situation which was causing these spells to recur over and over.

''You're barking up the wrong tree, doctor,'' she said. ''There is nothing bothering me. I have a wealthy husband, a lovely home, servants, a fine young son who is musically talented. . . I have nothing to worry about. In fact there is nothing I want that I could not have.''

I said, ''I bet that if I were in your house for an hour or two I'd find out what is causing your migraines.''

''Wonderful, come to my house, we would be delighted to have you as a guest,'' she said. So the next time I was in her city on a speaking engagement, my wife and I visited her together. The woman served us tea and after a while my patient's mother-in-law joined us and she was something! She was what I would call a *professional beauty*. Her dress was meticulous and she was perfectly groomed. I am sure she spent most of her time making herself look beautiful and for her age, she was very successful. The contrast between her and my patient, who was a sincere but rather plain-looking woman was considerable. My patient looked like a woman who spent her time trying to make a comfortable home for her family and not being totally successful. Then the son joined us and his mother looked embarrassed. Knowing his father was head of his own large corporation and having been told he wanted the boy to follow in his footsteps, I was beginning to see possible sources of some of the problems.

Then the husband arrived home from the office and what

does he do but go up to his mother, hug her and kiss her and tell her she is beautiful. He hardly looked at his wife if you can imagine . . . no wonder she had migraines. Then the son went over and started to play the piano without saying a word and the father got real mad at him. Just before we left he said to his wife, "Oh, by the way, I have two of our leading attorneys from New York working on the reorganization of the company and they are coming to dinner." It was almost six o'clock by that time and I could tell she was annoyed.

The next day the husband called at my hotel as he wanted to speak to me privately. He wanted to know what I could do for his wife's migraines. He told me he had spent thousands of dollars and he felt badly that she had to suffer so much.

I told him there was nothing I could do for his wife's migraines. "But there are a few things you can do," I said. "First of all, get your mother out of there. Get her an apartment of her own."

"Yes, I've thought of that," he said. "I know how it distresses my wife. All right, I'll do it. I'll see that she moves out. . . that will be fine."

"And apparently your son is a cause of aggravation between you," I said. "He's old enough to be in a boarding school you know."

"Well, that would suit me just fine too." the man said.

"You must talk it over with your wife and convince her that these changes are best for everyone and let her know that you care about her. I would suggest that the next time you have attorneys in from New York that you take them and your wife out to dinner."

Apparently the man saw the light and his wife has been writing to me every Christmas and sometimes in between telling me how grateful she is. The migraines left her immediately and they have a very happy life.

LONELINESS IS NOT A DISEASE

I imagine that some people, when they read here of the many patients whom I could not hope to cure entirely of their disease may be wondering "Why then go to a doctor?" Often it is well to go because, first of all, they can probably get some help physically and frequently a tremendous amount of help emotionally. Physicians have such a great opportunity in seeing hundreds of patients and learning how they cope with various illnesses and the emotional problems that accompany them that often they can pass on information from one to another. Most importantly, the support and understanding of a well-trained and sympathetic physician can be of much help and comfort to a troubled person. Many times I have seen an hour's chat work almost a transformation in the life of a nervous, depressed or frightened patient.

A while ago one of the saddest women I ever saw came to see me. I could not find anything physically wrong with her. Later I learned that for years she had worked alone as a bookkeeper, only occasionally seeing her boss who signed papers but did not talk with her. On retirement, she simply returned to her room where she lived completely alone. Her physical problems were really no more than those which naturally come with growing older, but being alone with nothing to look forward to caused her to be overly concerned. It took great courage for her to move to an apartment complex where there were many others her age and an even greater effort to force herself to be outgoing enough to make friends. Once this was accomplished however she told me she felt better, was more active and was enjoying life more than she ever had before.

I can recall many women who were cured of a bad neurosis by getting them to become active in helping the Y.W.C.A., their church, the Salvation Army or one of the many other worthwhile organizations which so desperately need help.

There are so many who make time their greatest enemy. In

the early adult years there never seems to be enough time and in the later years after retirement, too much time. It is a wise and healthy person who learns to use time well.

I just received a letter from a lovely woman whom I saw thirty-six years ago. She turned to me for comfort when her husband had a big stroke. She said the sympathetic chat we had then helped to direct her life at an important time and did her a world of good. Often I have helped largely by listening to patients, helping them to make up their wavering minds about whether or not to obtain a divorce or making other large decisions in life. Many said they were so much happier knowing that someone like me knew of their problem and had sympathy, respect and even some affection for them. A doctor also can help the very nervous person by giving medicine that will quiet nerves and relieve pain and insomnia, allowing the mind and the body sufficient time to relax and heal so that life's problems can be worked out.

My good friends, Dr. and Mrs. Maxwell Berry of Atlanta have devoted much time and effort to the founding of a village where they are bringing together the intellectually handicapped from eighteen years of age and up and the active retired volunteers who teach and help in a mutually rewarding relationship. Annandale Village, as it is called, is located within the town of Suwanee thirty miles outside of Atlanta, in a lovely setting with a hundred acres of land and a beautiful lake. At present the cottages house only the handicapped. The retired volunteers come on a daily basis, but as funding becomes available they look forward to the day when the retired volunteers can also have living accommodations within the village. The results of bringing together the needs and knowledge, physical services and companionship of these two very different groups has proved to be rewarding to all concerned. Long lasting bonds of friendship, caring, respect and trust are constantly being formed.

Many people have learned that happiness and health can often be found by getting and keeping many friends, and by helping other people who need help.

Remember. . .

Anger, depression, fright, sorrow, shock or trauma do exert tremendous influences upon your physical body.

Uncontrollable emotion can make you severely, physically ill. If unchecked, the eventual result may be fatal.

Your doctor needs to know what emotional state preceded your illness in order to diagnose and treat you effectively.

Instead of living with a nagging fear that something may be wrong with you, consult your doctor and find out for sure. Many times simply having his confirmation and assurance of your good health will make you well because it may be only the dread of disease that is making you sick.

Sometimes it is necessary to make a difficult choice which will change your entire life, but if such a decision is costing you your good health, the sooner you make that change the better off you will be.

The best prescription for maintaining good health is active, productive use of time and meaningful relationships with others.

Chapter Five

Are Those Tests Necessary?

Don't think the doctor is ignorant or careless if he advises you not to go ahead with a long and expensive examination; this action usually means not that he is careless, but rather that he hates to waste your time and money. He knows that it is almost always useless to search for a localized cause of high blood pressure, sick headaches, the jitters or nervous breakdown. It is useless to do much examining when a man is obviously suffering from old age, little strokes, rheumatoid arthritis or a widely scattered cancer.

In spite of the fact that every year more and more wonderful laboratory, x-ray and other tests are being used in the diagnoses of disease, I have to keep asking some of my young medical friends to remember that still a few diseases can be better diagnosed with the eyes and ears, and sometimes that is the best way of diagnosing them. Certainly it is the most economical way.

One day the president of one of America's greatest companies called me. He told me of one of his vice-presidents who had been an active and energetic figure in the company for years, but who for the past two months had been totally ineffective. The man had been sent to four well-known physicians, each of whom reported he could find nothing physically wrong with him.

I agreed to see him and an appointment was made. As the man came through my door, I was surprised to see he was leaning heavily on his wife's arm and his face was vacuous and lethargic.

I asked his wife "Did this terrible change come over your husband suddenly?" She said, "Yes, one evening he fell out of his chair while reading the paper. Ever since he has been so different I hardly know him."

Obviously the man had had a little stroke which four reputable doctors had failed to diagnose by examinations and tests, but none had thought his appearance strange for an executive or bothered to ask his wife what had happened.

Perhaps medical professors are now teaching their students to diagnose more often with their eyes, ears and touch. I have frequently suggested to deans of medical schools to *show* sick patients to their students and to teach them to diagnose some diseases with their eyes.

I well remember a man whom I once saw who lost his life because he trusted more to the diagnosis made by a bit of electronic apparatus than to the diagnosis made by two widely-experienced physicians who talked to him about his symptoms and even observed one of his attacks.

It happened one day while I was in a store; I was asked to see a customer whom the clerks thought was dying of a heart attack. When I saw the man I agreed that from his ghastly appearance, his fast irregular pulse, his frightened face, his shortness of breath and his statement of severe pain in the middle of his chest, he was having a bad heart attack. But soon he came out of it.

He told me he had had a number of such attacks. He admitted that since they started coming he had lost strength, he could not walk as fast as he used to and he had to climb stairs very slowly. Any overexertion would bring chest pain.

But he said, "This trouble is not with my heart because a heart specialist found my electrocardiogram (results of a test for diagnosing abnormalities of heart action) normal." That satisfied the doctor that the patient's heart must be normal.

I took the man a few doors away to a friend of mine, who, in puzzling cases, used the "Master Two-Step Test" devised by my old friend, the late Dr. Master of New York City. It consists of having the patient walk up two steps to a platform and down two steps on the other side (a form of exercise) and seeing if that makes a notable change in the electrocardiogram. The doctor soon had to stop the test because the patient immediately went into one of his painful coronary attacks. We agreed that the man had a bad heart; to make matters worse, he had very little reserve strength. We warned him that he had better be careful not to further overstrain his heart.

But the man insisted there was no reason to curtail his activities. The heart specialist he had seen earlier taught in a university, he trusted his electrocardiograms, and the man was therefore going to accept his specialist's opinion. Only a few days later the patient went on a business trip to a distant city and upon arriving there, died of one of his attacks.

Violent tempers and unwarranted anxieties

Persons who have spells of emotional storm such as great fear or nervousness for no apparent reason and more particularly people who frequently "fly off the handle," should have an electroencephalogram (a reading of the brain waves) test. There are some ten million people living in America who are suffering from a form of non-convulsive epilepsy. In my last ten years of practice I found hundreds of such people and was delighted to be able to relieve their suffering, usually overnight, with the wonderful medication available for treating epilepsy.

One of those was a young man, the grandson of one of my colleagues. He had a long history of maladjustment and difficulties in school; he took out his frustrations on everyone around him. Long before, the family had practically given up all hope of him ever amounting to anything. I was asked by my friend to come to the house and was shocked upon entering the boy's room to see him haul off and punch the wall with his bare fist which was swollen and bleeding. He insisted that he wasn't really mad at anyone, he was *just mad.*

I talked to him at length about his feelings and then had the proper tests made. They came back with a definite confirmation of the epilepsy I had suspected although the young man had never in his life suffered a convulsion. When given the medication he was like a different person and has been in control of his emotions ever since. He graduated from a fine university and the last I heard of him was when I received as a gift a copy of a book he had recently published on archeology.

Confirming a hunch

Once I saw a woman who, while traveling in Europe, began to suffer from sweats, shivers and shakes that seemed to suggest a very severe menopause. She had been seen by well-respected professors in Vienna, Berlin, Paris and London and all agreed she was having a violent menopause.

Her symptoms, which of course were all common in menopause, reminded me of the work of a very able woman chemist who was showing through chemical tests that similar symptoms were produced by a little yellow tumor in the adrenal gland (above the kidney). I sent her to the Mayo Clinic where the test was made and she did indeed have such a tumor. A surgeon there removed it and her symptoms were gone; the woman was immediately well.

Although chemical tests are invaluable in the making of many difficult diagnoses, still, a number of *possible causes* are missed by the doctor who does not look with great care and wisdom at the patient, taking into consideration the whole person, their way of life and a careful medical history. In this case I was encouraged to look further since this active and intelligent woman did not seem the type to be so totally incapacitated by menopause. It was not in keeping with her character.

Some tests you can make yourself (with your doctor's approval)

I have been able to give complete relief to hundreds of people with chronic indigestion by finding that they had a food allergy, and then isolating the offending food. I use techniques which I like much more than the skin tests that are often used.

If the person has *spells* of indigestion with good digestion in between, I have him/her keep a diary of the *unusual* foods eaten just before a spell. If the person's indigestion comes every day, then for two days I put him/her on my *elimination* diet consisting of *nothing but* lamb, rice, butter and canned pears. If on this he/she is comfortable, then every two days I add a new food and the reaction of each food is noted. In most cases this works very well and it is not difficult to tell when the allergy-producing food is introduced into the diet. Interestingly enough, for many people the most frequent offender is onions, and the second is milk!

Home detective work

I frequently employ "home detective work" since I find the results more accurate and of course it is certainly more economical. This is particularly true of strange allergies since those tests start with the most common allergy-producing products and if it were something unusual, a great amount of testing is required before the dilemma is solved.

For instance, I saw an asthmatic woman who was constantly ill in her *own* home and who occasionally had spells when she visited *other* homes. Of particular interest was the fact that when she stayed at the home of her parents the problem immediately cleared up. To further confuse the situation she was ill at home but when she came to Rochester to the Mayo Clinic she promptly lost her asthmatic symptoms. By coincidence her husband happened to be a builder. I asked him to take a look at the construction of the various houses and compare the materials in the homes where she had attacks of asthma with those where she was free of it. Her husband was astounded when he learned that their own home and others which brought on the symptoms had areas of unpainted beaverboard, while her parents' home and other buildings where she was well (including the Mayo Clinic) had no unpainted beaverboard in their construction. He promptly painted or varnished the unfinished beaverboard surfaces in their home and we heard no more complaints of asthma from his wife.

I recall another patient, a farmer, who came complaining of an occasional spell of asthma. During his Mayo Clinic examination, tests showed that the cause was not the foods which he commonly ate, nor was it the ordinary surroundings of his home. I asked him to go home and report exactly what he did just before each attack. In a few days he reported that he became ill when he drove his car into the city. I told him to try it again but not to go all the way into the city, only to the edge of the city and return home. He came back to report that he got the attack anyway so it was not due to something in the city.

Then I became suspicious of his car and suggested he go to the city by bus or the neighbor's car but he reported back that it didn't make any difference. Any time he went to the city by whatever method of transporation, he became ill.

Later he phoned in great excitement to say, "When I went into the city today I took a narrow country road and I had no trouble." So I said, "Explore the highway that you usually use and see if you can find what it is there that gets you." This he did and soon found it was swampelder, a plant which grew near the highway, that caused his violent asthmatic reaction.

Keeping a record

I have seen many cases in which a patient had gallstones which were not producing the symptoms commonly associated with "gallbladder attack." For years I had spells of abdominal pain which for a time I thought were due to emotion because they often came after I had spoken at a big banquet. But because many such spells also came when I was quiet at home, I knew there had to be another cause.

Then I thought of allergy and decided to keep a record of the foods eaten before my painful spells. As you may be well aware, chicken is a favorite entree for banquets, and in my case it was frequently served in our home also. I soon found that each time I had a spell of abdominal pain, it was after I had eaten chicken or chicken soup. My digestion has been almost perfect since I stopped eating chicken. But interestingly, I am the only member of my family to have this allergy to chicken. My two sons once had a chicken-eating contest, during which they both consumed huge quantities of the bird (they were teen-agers then). I don't think they even had stomachaches!

Remember...

Your doctor's decision of whether or not tests are necessary will depend upon *your* case and your condition. Sometimes the obvious facts are a better guide than tests.

Persons who are plagued with emotional storms, bad temper or unwarranted fear or nervousness should have an electroencephalogram taken to determine if they have non-convulsive epilepsy.

Some recurring illnesses can be tested by the patient at home better and more economically than in the laboratory by keeping a record of foods eaten in cases of chronic indigestion or by listing exposure to unusual plants or products in cases of asthmatic attack.

Chapter Six

Is That Surgery Necessary?

The decision to submit to elective surgery is difficult and requires the advice of medical professionals. However, each situation must be considered individually. I imagine most people, having been told by a doctor that they need an operation, would feel in some danger if they did not have it.

When, in 1926 an x-ray man, in a routine examination, found that I had gallstones, my doctor friends said, "Go get operated on." But I said, "I will not bother my gallstones until they bother me." They haven't bothered me for a moment and now, fifty years later, I still have them.

In 1950 I was told that my prostate gland was twice the normal size. I asked my friend Dr. Thompson, then perhaps the ablest prostate surgeon in the world, if he wanted to operate on me. He said, "Walter, if you weren't my friend I might be talked into operating on you, but you are my friend and your prostate is not bothering you a particle, so I won't operate on you!" I am still grateful to him for helping me to avoid that needless surgery because that prostate gland still hasn't bothered me, even after all those years.

Of course if an operable cancer were found, your doctor would insist it be operated on right away. It would be very important to your health to take his advice and to have the surgery as quickly as possible. But I can tell you from experience, if a trusted and able doctor says "You don't have to have that operation now; don't have it until the organ annoys you," take his advice. You will save time, money and suffering, and it is possible that it never will bother you.

Chronic Appendicitis

Sometimes I have wondered if there is such a disease as chronic appendicitis. In fact, for several months I conducted a survey by questioning carefully every patient who came into my office with a scar over his/her appendix area. If the operation had been for a "chronic appendicitis" I asked with particular care what had been the result, what relief had been experienced. I found that only a very few patients believed they had been helped. Those who were helped were usually those who, apparently shortly before the operation, had had a severe flare-up of acute appendicitis.

Gallstones

In scores of cases when friendly young colleagues of mine had examined patients with x-rays and found gallstones, they naturally assumed that their work was done; the diagnosis was made and all that was left to do was turn the patient over to a surgeon for removal of the stones. Although such medical men may eventually become fine doctors, their lack of experience in recognizing symptomless gallstones is unfortunate for the patient. Often I would be called in because the patient had been referred to me by their hometown doctor.

Time and again I would learn that the patient had never had any pain or indigestion due to the gallstones and I would say of the surgeon, "I hope you do not operate, because removing those stones will not help a particle and you might make matters worse."

In pursuing the case we almost always found that the cause of the problem had nothing to do with the symptomless gallstones.

Today in some hospitals, every bit of tissue that is removed by a surgeon is studied by a "tissue committee," and if a surgeon has too high a record of taking out normal appendices or gall bladders, he is refused the use of the operating rooms.

Improper information can deceive a surgeon into operating

After I had seen thousands of patients who neglected to give me accurate and honest answers to my questions I felt a great need to convince people how terribly that sort of thing can hurt them. In many cases it has deceived the physician and the surgeon into performing operations which were both needless and useless.

I think most layman should see that when the illness followed immediately after some great trauma, great annoyance, great sorrow, or great loss of a loved one, the illness was probably due to that disaster. Why on earth conceal that fact from the doctor? It can result only in his wasting time, vainly, trying to find some other cause. And it is in such cases especially that if he should find something like silent gallstones, he may think, "Here we have the cause of the illness, so we will operate."

Sometimes the operation will do more harm than good

I will never forget the wonderful but very nervous woman of forty who came to me with her husband who was very concerned about her. She had a definite fibroma (fibrous tumor) of her uterus. In chatting with her I learned that she was so nervous as to be on the edge of a psychosis. I said, "No operation for her. An operation might throw her into a mental hospital!" They were tremendously happy and grateful that I forbade operating.

Knowing that she did not have to face surgery helped her nervous condition tremémdously. I hear from her at least every Christmas. She enjoys good health except for her decided nervousness.

A good example of what many patients do, unwisely

A forty-seven-year-old unmarried business woman came to me complaining of spells of severe diarrhea that had been afflicting her for six years. She insisted that there were no severe mental strains in her life. Knowing that some people get spells of diarrhea because of panics, I asked her if she had them; also I asked if she had any mentally disturbed relatives, but she vigorously insisted she did not. Unfortunately, an x-ray man found a big pouch on the side of her duodenum. Fearing that stagnation of food in that pouch could be causing the woman's spells, I turned her over to a surgeon who removed it. However, we soon learned that operation did not alleviate the problem.

When the operation did not help, I was ashamed and expected her to be angry with me, but she wasn't. In fact she came back hoping for another operation. I took her history over again and found that she had not told me the most important point which was that a number of her spells of diarrhea had come when she had thoughts of suicide, which she confessed happened when she had brief periods of psychotic depression. Other spells came with panics when she feared she was going insane and then came the story of some of her mentally ill ancestors. I asked why she had denied having insane relatives and she said because she did not want to be turned over to a psychiatrist.

This woman would not have had a useless operation if some concerned relative had come with her and told me the truth about her psychotic panics and her insane ancestry.

Get Yourself a Lawyer

One day a woman came into my office and said, "Don't waste time giving me examinations and medicines. . . I am too sick for that sort of thing. Only an operation can cure me now, so go ahead and get a surgeon." Actually, this was not an unusual occurrence. It happened to me many times over the years.

As was my custom I told the woman I would have to examine her first and soon I was telling her that her symptoms were very definitely indicative of a neurosis after a bad shock. I said "Please tell me what happened that upset you so badly."

She became angry and left my office. A few days later I received a very unpleasant letter from her telling me that she had found a surgeon who was going to do a hysterectomy. Some time went by and meanwhile I learned from her sister that she had indeed had several traumatic experiences. First was her husband's almost fatal stroke. Immediately after that she learned that in his will he was leaving most of his fortune, not to her, but to the grown children born to his previous wife. No wonder she had become ill!

Three months passed and then a very humble letter came saying that the operation, performed in her weak state, had resulted in her having to go to a mental hospital for several months.

Think how much suffering and money she could have saved herself had she believed me when I told her that her uterus was normal. If only she had told me the truth, I would have sent her to a good lawyer! He would have been better trained to handle her case than a surgeon.

Remember. . .

Your doctor or specialist will let you know when surgery is essential.

Avoid elective surgery unless it is absolutely necessary. If an organ doesn't bother you, don't bother it.

Doctors can be misled into operating unnecessarily when they find silent gallstones or are told of symptoms which indicate acute appendicitis and you withhold the vital information that might otherwise explain your true condition.

Chapter Seven

A Word to the Doctor

We used to call it *bedside manner.* "The attitude and conduct of a doctor in the presence of a patient, intended to inspire confidence," according to *The American Heritage Dictionary.* The attitude and conduct of a doctor does indeed influence the patient/doctor relationship, and it also influences to a large degree the success of maintaining general health as well as the diagnosis and treatment of a particular illness.

Recently I was appalled to read that the average length of time of an office call was seven minutes. Allowing time for the examination, I do not understand how a physician could obtain much more than an overview of his patient in only seven minutes. Certainly seven minutes it not sufficient to discuss even briefly any concerns the patient may have beyond the specific problem of the moment. It is important to make a brief analysis of the whole person, to inquire in a friendly and interested manner "How are things going with you?" Such a concerned inquiry will usually prompt the patient to voice his/her anxieties.

Unfortunately, patients have also been programmed not to take up too much of the doctor's time and are inhibited by seeing a waiting room filled with impatient people. A doctor can control this by allowing a realistic amount of time for each patient's visit. A physician needs to take a look at his particular practice from time to time. It is difficult for a doctor to turn new patients away, especially as he becomes known for his ability and is sought out by many people for help. However, if his schedule is overcrowded, he will do his regular patients a favor, and better serve the needs of new patients who call for an appointment as well, by referring the overflow to another doctor, perhaps an able man just getting his practice established. Then *all* will receive the services of a competent physician who has the proper motivation and who can take the time to give them the proper attention.

Sometimes even when a doctor does make every attempt to learn the personal facts surrounding a patient's problem, he is unsuccessful; often because of this hesitancy on the part of patients to take up the doctor's time with what they think are personal problems not related to their illness. Several times over the years I learned of instances when a patient told all kinds of troubles to a total stranger he met in my waiting room or sometimes to my nurse or receptionist but not to me. The case that still sticks most vividly in my mind is the first one and the reason I probably remember it so well is because it so shocked me.

There were two men whom I had been seeing for some time and occasionally they were both in my waiting room at the same time. Being congenial fellows, they had struck up a conversation even though strangers.

The one fellow had come to me complaining of what he insisted was a bad gall bladder; he wanted me to get a surgeon to remove it. But he did not have the symptoms which would indicate that removing his gall bladder would help him so I would not do that. I could see that the man was a bundle of nerves and he told me he could not sleep properly and that his stomach was bothering him. The man was terribly on edge. I told him "You have symptoms of anxiety and neurosis and there must be a situation which is causing all this distress." But my patient kept talking about his gall bladder, insisting there was no problem in his life, at work, or with his family that could possibly be creating all this trouble.

As he left I was still shaking my head and feeling a bit frustrated when the other gentleman who had been sitting in the waiting room off-handedly remarked, "A person doesn't know how lucky he is until he hears another man's problems. Boy, I'm sure glad I don't have that fellow's troubles!"

I was surprised, of course, and asked him if he would mind telling me since the other patient had not indicated there was any secret about it. So the man proceeded to tell me. It seemed he owned and operated quite a large business and for some reason was being sued for a substantial amount of money. It looked as though his life savings would be completely depleted and that he might even lose the business. He was terribly angry and upset with the people who were suing him and lay awake nights worrying about what was going to happen. In fact he was so upset he couldn't even eat.

The next time the man came in for an appointment concerning his gall bladder I opened the conversation with, "Well, how's business?" and sure enough with a little encouragement he finally told me the whole story. It honestly had not occurred to the man that this was what was making him sick. I suggested that he talk to his attorney and see if it would be possible to settle the case out of court. In the meantime I gave him a prescription for a mild sedative that would enable his mind and body to get some rest. A few days later he called me, absolutely elated. It seemed that the plaintiff was more than willing to get the matter settled without going to court and for a price that was much lower than my patient had anticipated. Once the matter was settled he soon forgot about his gall bladder and resumed his normal healthy life.

Another man I kept out of the hands of surgeons for

years. He had a slight ulcer which was usually kept under control through proper diet and normally it caused him very little discomfort. He was a professor of chemistry and had invented a procedure using a chemical in an industrial process. Every so often a new company would agree to take over the procedure, and sometimes the material they were using it on would be of a different composition and then the chemical wouldn't work.

They would call him and tell him his product was "no darn good" and that he "could come and get it."

Every time this happened his ulcer would flare up and he would have a terrible time with his stomach. This would continue until he had made the necessary tests and changed the formula of his invention so that it would work on the material the company was using. Once this was done, everything, particularly his health, would return to normal. I am still uncertain whether the man eventually learned not to get so upset or if perhaps he perfected the chemical to the point where it would work on any material. In any event, I do know that it was never necessary for him to be operated on for that ulcer.

Another patient dealt in antiques and for many years had a store near my office. I would stop in from time to time and purchase something from him for a gift. Much of his stock was shipped to him by his brother in London.

One year, the first week in December, he came to me with a whole list of aches and pains. I couldn't find anything physically wrong with the man but soon learned that he was really worried. He told me he depended heavily on his Christmas sales as the difference between good profit and serious loss each year. His brother had sent his entire Christmas stock in one shipment which should have arrived a month or six weeks earlier but the express company was unable to trace it. Days were passing quickly and if he did not receive it, not only would he be wiped out, but his brother would suffer great loss also. As it turned out it did finally arrive. It was so late that he did not do as well as he had hoped, but both his business and his health eventually recovered.

When the same man came to me in a similar state of anxiety with symptoms of nervous distress about a year later I was smart enough to ask how things were going at the antique store. My question obviously distressed him even more. This time he told me that business was better than ever but that he had lost the lease on his building and would be forced to move. This was a great problem for him. I suggested that the sooner he faced his problem, found a new location and "got on with it," the better he would feel. True to history, as soon as he was settled in his new location he was fine again.

Of course, a doctor's life would be an easy one if all cases were so simple. What I am trying to stress here however is the importance of helping the patient to feel at ease, confident that his physician wants to know what is on his patient's mind and how that might be affecting his health.

Ask the right questions. . . avoid the wrong words

A doctor must learn to carefully select his words so that they are meaningful within the patient's realm of experience. In previous chapters we have talked about having the patient show the doctor, with his hand, the area of his body to which he is referring. Also, a doctor can ask leading questions in simple lay terms which will draw the patient into further explanation. Often I found questions of a personal nature about the patient's job or home life would bring forth a wealth of information.

It is also wise to avoid using words which have a stigma attached to them and which may cause an unnecessary unpleasant reaction in the patient. A good example of this is the word "insanity," today the terms "mental illness" and "mental health" are used instead.

In trying to confirm a suspicion of a tendency toward inherited mental illness I may ask a patient if his father was a kindly and well-respected man. If the patient answers "No, he was an alcoholic good-for-nothing whom I despised," that tells me quite alot. Other questions, such as, "Is your family close? Do you see your brothers and sisters often?" may bring such responses as, "My brothers are no good," "My only sister left home and we never heard from her again," "They have no use for the rest of the family," or some other indication of mental or emotional problems.

Epilepsy, a disease on which I spent a great deal of time in research and treatment, is another which patients wish to avoid discussing. Many people act as though they believe that epilepsy is contagious though, it certainly is not. However, while I worked in the gastroenterology section of Mayo Clinic many non-convulsive epileptics came to me, usually because of an abdominal discomfort, but never because of a convulsion. Usually they had one or more epileptic relatives and might well have suspected what was causing them so much discomfort, but because of the terrible and entirely unjustified stigma attached to epilepsy many preferred not to be sure about it. However, if I had a severe nervous illness I would pray that it was epilepsy because it can be so greatly relieved with proper medication. But here again, the doctor must be *extremely tactful* in choosing the right words in order to get an accurate family and medical history.

The value of a doctor's experience

An internist will soon acquire skill in recognizing the visual symptoms in the appearances of patients with various illnesses. For example, when an attractive and trim-bodied woman walked quickly into my office and shaded her eyes from the sun coming in through my window, I had my first clue of migraine. With migraine her eyes might be quite sensitive to the bright sunlight. Over the years I had learned that it was more than likely that a person who suffers from migraines tends to walk and move quickly, has an unusually alert mind, and is almost never overweight.

Of course, as soon as one makes such a statement one remembers the case that was the exception to the rule. I once had a patient who had the symptoms of migraine but her case puzzled me because my findings didn't seem to ring true. Watching her walk rapidly down a corridor one day it finally dawned on me that she was obviously overweight and that was causing me to doubt my diagnosis. I called her aside and asked if she had gained the weight since she became ill and how it had happened. She told me that she had indeed put on more than forty pounds. When she first became ill her hometown doctor, suspecting that she was suffering from a gastric ulcer, encouraged her to eat quantities of bland foods whenever she felt discomfort, which of course was most of the time. So I was satisfied that my sleuthing had uncovered the cause of the exception to the rule.

Noticing the obvious

It is of tremendous importance for a physician to learn enough about a patient to determine whether or not his appearance and his symptoms are in keeping with his established character. Once, for about a year, I traveled about the country lecturing to groups of physicians on the significance of "gravy on the vest."

This came about because I became aware that many able physicians seldom seemed to notice or realize the significance of seeing an elderly man of refinement and wealth who went out on the street or to an important appointment with gravy on his vest, soup on his tie, or who generally had a sudden lack of awareness of his appearance. My series of lectures was the result of my strong feelings that doctors should recognize such things as clues to little strokes.

Sudden aging of the face and odd behavior are other clues. There are many little strokes which an aging person can have over the years which can damage such a tiny part of the brain that a person can have thirty of them and lose only some of his memory, his ability to walk up a hill comfortably or his ability to run down stairs.

I once asked a brain pathologist what happened to the brains of patients who had suffered little strokes. He showed me photographs of brains with little black spots here and there. He said they were tiny blood clots in a blood vessel. He had tried to interest doctors in those spots but had often failed and finally gave up trying.

In most cases if the doctor asks a member of the family if the change came suddenly they will say "Yes, one day he/she fell . . . became dizzy and disoriented . . . seemed like a total stranger . . . ," etc.

One can be suspicious when a man whose face is apathetic, dull and uninterested lists his occupation as a company executive. Frequently he will answer questions concerning his condition very poorly. In some cases I have noticed that a person with brain damage will walk peculiarly, often with very short steps.

In teaching my students to recognize physical symptoms in patients I often tell them of a man of forty who came to me. He said he had suffered all his life with spells of depression, wooziness and a violent temper. His facial skin was somewhat thickened and brownish as one sees occasionally in elderly epileptics. I asked him if he had ever had a convulsion and he said "No." However when I inquired if any of his relatives had epilepsy he told me of his brother who had a bad case of it.

It is sad that more doctors do not make a real effort to uncover cases of mild epilepsy in their patients. Petit mal, psychomotor and Jacksonian (mild epilepsies without a big convulsion) are fairly common, but so few seem to know of those mild epilepsies in which the person is only very nervous, often depressed and easily enraged. I became particularly interested in this phenomenon around 1940 and soon found four hundred cases of mild epilepsy among my patients. Not a single one had had his nervousness diagnosed correctly! After much study of the literature on several types of mild epilepsy, and after much analysis of 274 of my cases, I wrote a book entitled *Nerves in Collision,* which further examines this little-known but widespread form of epilepsy.

Dr. Frederic Gibbs, the country's great expert on electroencephalograms has helped me greatly for twenty-five years. Dr. Gibbs tells me that for every epileptic he sees *with* convulsions, he sees ten *without.* And he is the sort of man whose statement I would never doubt. That means that if, as authorities say, there are over a million epileptics in this country, there must be over ten million who do not yet know what is wrong and that proper medication might work a miracle in their lives.

Constitutional inadequacy

In my early years of practice I began to see a few men and women who were cursed by one or several illnesses all the time for years. Some nervous people seem never to get permanently well. My impression is that those who have psychotic ancestors have the hardest time to get and stay well, and there have been times when I dreaded to try to treat them. Some do not seem to care to make a great effort and they do not seem to learn from experience. One can only treat their periodic storms and encourage them to work to control their emotions.

Medication

Another point I have learned to clarify with patients is exactly what medication a patient was taking, whether prescriptions from another doctor or "across-the-counter" remedies sold without prescription. I have had many patients who were cured simply by taking away medicine they had, rather than giving them another medicine.

Once I had a woman come to me who had gone to a series of doctors for a ringing in her right ear, but getting no relief. Finally she went to a doctor who insisted on knowing exactly how much of and every type of pill she was taking. When he learned that she was taking massive doses of a vitamin that had become popular through recent magazine articles, he told her to stop and see what happened. The ringing in her ear cleared up as soon as the overdose of vitamins cleared her body. Sometimes patients are badly hurt by taking too large a dose of some medicine or by continuing it for too long a time.

A careful doctor will give his patient explicit instruction along with the prescription. I found it was particularly necessary to do this for example in administering an antibiotic such as penicillin. Many patients will quit taking the medication the minute the symptoms clear up, frequently resulting in a prompt recurrence of the infection. It is wise to give prescriptions in realistic amounts, advising the patient to continue use until it is used up. This also helps to guard against "left over" medications which people often tend to try using for something else, or worse yet, for someone else.

Doctors, please remember . . .

Control the size of the practice so that sufficient time can be spent with each patient.

Direct the conversation so the patient will feel at ease and encouraged to talk about what is bothering him, within reason, of course. A doctor can control the conversation to learn the necessary facts while not allowing the patient to waste an excessive amount of time in idle chatter.

Have the patient show you with his hand the area of his body to which *he* is referring.

Choose words carefully in talking with a patient and avoid those which have a stigma attached. Be tactful.

Look for and learn to recognize the visual symptoms of specific illnesses.

Ask what medication the patient is taking; it may be doing more harm than good.

Prescribe your own medications with specific instructions for using them completely. Give only realistic amounts so left-overs do not accumulate in family medicine cabinets.

Chapter Eight

Where and How to Find the Right Doctor

Sometimes I have a twinge of conscience because I frequently advise readers to "go to a good physician or a good specialist," and I know that isn't as simple as it sounds. Many people have absolutely no idea how to go about finding a good physician or specialist. Without doubt, doing so is a very personal matter; it may be necessary to consult several before finding the physician with whom you feel comfortable. He or she should be someone whose judgment you trust and you should feel confident of his/her ability. He should be a person in whom you can confide. The rapport you establish with this very important person cannot be exaggerated; there may come a day when your very life may depend upon him. Beyond that, it is important that you then carefully follow his advice and instruction. It isn't enough simply to say to yourself, "He's probably right," and then do as he says only in a casual or haphazard manner.

It amazes me how little care people, even very sick people, take in finding a better-than-average physician. They seem to rely on hope and good luck, and will go to the man whose shingle they have seen because he is practicing over the neighborhood drugstore. Another source is hearing someone else, often a chance acquaintance, rave about a doctor who performed some fantastic cure, and then going to him without making any effort whatever to check on the man's education and qualifications. People may also be influenced to accept this method because they are concerned that a well-known specialist will be more expensive. In the long run, an expert who is able to examine, diagnose and treat them properly from the beginning will cost a good deal less than will going to several poorly-trained men who, over a long period of time, are still unable to make a diagnosis and who may continue to dispense medicine and treat without being of any real help to the patient. Many people do not recognize the need to look for a well-trained man; others assume that if a person uses initials after his name, he is without question qualified or he wouldn't be practicing.

Although medical societies and other groups within the medical profession go to great effort to keep available accurate records of qualified doctors, it is not always possible for them to keep track of those persons who are not registered with them. *Clinics* and *foundations*, most of which are entirely reputable, should, however, be checked out since some charlatans use the prestige value of these terms. A call to the office of the county medical society will determine very quickly if such clinics or foundations are reputable. Likewise, most doctors are well-trained, idealistic women and men who have made every effort to obtain the best medical education available and who continue to study and keep abreast of all new innovations in medicine and health care. They are truly concerned and compassionate, take the time and have the patience necessary to listen and learn everything there is to know about a patient which might be affecting the state of his or her physical and mental health. But, like all human beings, doctors can be good, bad or indifferent. I would particularly caution a patient concerning those who are indifferent.

Unfortunately there are also some few who made the mistake of getting into a profession for which they were not suited. One will find doctors with huge practices who have iron constitutions and work rapidly all day and half the night but do not really have the time to listen to the patient or to keep up with the advancements in medical knowledge. Such doctors tend to rely too heavily on extensive laboratory work and x-rays rather than paying attention to what the sick person is saying.

Frequently, the ablest physicians, with national reputations, limit their practices in order to have time for study, lecturing, writing and directing societies designed for furthering public health and medical advancement.

Although there are no specific guidelines to guarantee finding the right physician for you on your first attempt there are certainly some methods of going about it that are better than others.

You must first of all decide if you are looking for a family practitioner who will serve the medical needs of the entire family and who will send you to a specialist when he feels that is required. In many families today, members with specific problems go to different specialists. The children may go to a pediatrician; the wife or mother may depend on her obstetrician or gynecologist; and so on.

If you have a long-time and trusted physician you may wish to consult him before moving to a new location. He can help you in selecting the names of several competent persons who are practicing in the area of your new home. If he doesn't personally know anyone to recommend in that city, he most likely has access to the *Directory of Physicians* published by the American Medical Association and/or the *Directory of Medical Specialists* published by the American Board of Medical Specialties.

Both of these important volumes are generally available at the reference desk of any large public library or in the library of the county medical society. Locating the information you seek in these books is a relatively simple matter. The *Direc-*

tory of Physicians contains three volumes, the first being an alphabetical index of physicians and the second and third geographical registers. One can quickly look up the state and city and find a list of doctors practicing there. If the physician's last name is in bold face type it indicates that he is a member of the AMA. After the name and address there follows a series of code letters and numbers which refer back to an explanation in the front matter of the book indicating the year he was born, from what medical school and in what year he received his degree, the year he became licensed in the state in which he is now practicing, if he is certified as a specialist in a certain field, and any special societies of which he is a member.

The *Directory of Medical Specialists* lists only those physicians who are Certified by their national board after having passed thorough examination procedures. It also gives a brief personal biography of each person listed, including the medical schools he has attended, the degrees he has attained, graduate study, teaching positions he has held, and scientific organizations of which he is a member or from which he has received honors.

You may wish to consult the county medical society which is an excellent source of information. Your local telephone directory will list the medical societies in your area. Their lists will reflect all doctors who have met the society's qualifications which include their state license, a minimum length of practice, and approval by the board of directors of the society. They will generally not recommend only one particular physician but rather will provide the names of at least three doctors in the area where you live who are qualified in the field you specify. Questions you may wish to ask might include the name of the medical school where the doctor studied, where he had an internship and if he is on the staff of one or more of the local hospitals.

The person in charge will usually be happy to provide you

with as much information as possible but of course cannot express any opinion as to the capabilities of the physicians whose names he/she will give you. However, if you have been advised to go to a certain doctor and for any reason you feel that everything is not quite as it should be, the medical society will know if he has been suspended from the society, if he does indeed have the credentials he says he has, or in the case of an extreme "bad actor" has served a term in prison for selling drugs illegally or some other unprofessional conduct.

Also, the American Medical Association, 535 North Dearborn, Chicago, Illinois, 60610, has extensive files on known medical imposters and quacks; should you find yourself distrustful of a particular "doctor" or medical facility, a letter to the AMA offices should provide the information you seek.

The American Academy of Family Physicians, 1740 West 92nd Street, Kansas City, Missouri, 64114, will also provide information which should be helpful to anyone seeking an able family doctor in their community. They have a roster of general practitioners who are actively taking refresher courses to continually improve their knowledge. Family Practice has now been accepted as a medical specialty and will be included in future publications of the *Directory of Medical Specialists.* The certifying board requires specialists in family practice to pass current examinations every six years to be included in their roster.

In Chapter Eleven I have listed a number of health organizations, which, in addition to their other services, may provide helpful information concerning specialists available in your area in a variety of fields.

Should your residence be in a metropolitan area where there is a good medical school, it too may be another simple and valuable source of locating a competent doctor. I would suggest calling the Dean's secretary and requesting the names of one or two instructors who might provide the necessary information. Also there are often special hospitals or institutes affiliated with the school which treat certain diseases. A telephone call to the office of the director of one of these should provide a valuable lead.

Frequently, medical schools also have provision for examination and treatment by members of their own staff, and of course, in such institutions one is assured of a thorough examination by well-qualified doctors. Some medical schools even provide care at reduced rates if one is unable to pay the full cost.

If you are located near, or have a preference for, a certain hospital, it may be the best place to look for the right doctor. By calling the hospital administrative offices they will be able to tell you the names of the physicians on their staff and although, here again, cannot recommend a particular doctor, may give you the names of several practitioners at the hospital who have offices in your immediate vicinity. Or, you could go to the hospital of your choice and ask to see one of the resident physicians. Upon learning of your effort to locate a physician he may be willing to say who on the staff or in the city would be a good man to see.

Still another source which many people do not think of, is the large casualty insurance companies. They know competent physicians and specialists whom they consider to be tops in their field and upon whom they call when they need expert opinions.

Possibly one of the most expedient and successful ways in which to go about finding a doctor is to ask advice from a personal acquaintance whose judgment you respect and who is familiar within the community. Personal knowledge and referral is certainly preferable to hearsay. When you move to a new area you will meet people through your employment and neighborhood, or get acquainted through a church, lodge, service club group, etc. As you make friends and learn to rely on various members of the community you will find people eager to help you get settled in your new surroundings as quickly and completely as possible.

So there are quite a number of avenues to pursue when trying to locate the right doctor. Actually, a combination of these methods would most likely insure the best results; a referral from a health organization or a recommendation by a trusted acquaintance, followed by a routine check of the available directories and local medical societies.

In making your initial appointment with a new doctor it is wise to ask the nurse or receptionist to schedule sufficient time to allow discussion of any questions you may wish to ask him. I have known particularly popular and competent doctors who limit the number of new patients they take in order to be certain their regular patients are provided with as much time as they need. This is certainly to the doctor's credit since you would expect him, if he were your doctor, to expend the time and effort which your health necessarily requires.

PROTOCOL

In establishing a good relationship with your doctor and his staff you should not hesitate to inquire about his policies and procedures. There is nothing more frustrating that becoming suddenly ill, or having a child or other member of your family become sick, perhaps on a weekend or very late at night, and finding it difficult to locate your doctor or to learn from an answering service that he is out of town. Doctors do take vacations, go out of town, have personal lives and personal needs. However, all reputable physicians also know their patients may have need for medical care in their absence and make provision for it to the best of their ability. Usually another doctor with a similar practice who is on the staff of the same hospital will be designated by your doctor to provide emergency care in his absence.

It is also good to know whether or not your doctor will make house calls in the event of an emergency when it seems advisable not to take the patient from the house. Also, a patient must make allowances when a routine appointment is interrupted or postponed due to an emergency of another patient. That will certainly indicate that the doctor's time and attention would be with you in the event of an emergency.

Should you, the patient, feel you would like to have a second medical opinion from a specialist in a certain field and your doctor has not suggested it, by all means discuss it with him. No reputable and competent physician would object to or be in the least offended by such a request. He will probably ask if you have someone in mind or if you would like him to recommend someone. It is entirely possible that he feels a second opinion might be advisable, if for no other reason than to relieve the patient's concern, but he may not have suggested it himself for fear the expense would cause a financial hardship.

Quite often the family physician and the specialist will consult together over their findings and the regular family doctor will keep track of the overall situation with the specialist. A friend of mine once told me how her family doctor had given her the name of a surgeon when her little daughter's tonsils repeatedly became infected. She had taken the girl to the surgeon who examined her and made arrangements with the hospital for the tonsilectomy to be performed very early in the morning a couple of weeks later. The surgeon also examined the child again on the day when she was admitted to the hospital—the day before surgery was scheduled. The parents assumed that the child's care was now completely in the hands of the surgeon.

They were surprised to see their family doctor walk through the hospital corridor at 5:30 a.m. the morning of the operation but since he seemed to be in a hurry they did not speak to him. However, when their daughter came out of the anesthetic they were delighted to learn that she had been greatly comforted by their family doctor who held her hand and chatted with her as she lay on the gurney, waiting her turn in surgery. Even though she was under sedation, the one thing she remembered was that her own familiar friend and doctor had been there beside her.

Should you wish to change doctors

If for some reason you find you do not have confidence in your doctor, then by all means you should find one with whom you do feel comfortable. This presents a serious problem to many people, the main reason simply being that they do not understand the situation or how to approach it.

Unfortunately it is something that has not been discussed openly because many doctors do not wish to cause annoyance to patients or to interfere with their getting good medical service. However, if you stop to think for a moment, as is the case in any other profession, doctors in a city must have some code of politeness to each other if they are to avoid misunderstanding, hurt feelings and the breakup of personal friendships. If they can work happily together, it is the patient who will benefit most.

There is definitely an etiquette which should be followed either in changing doctors or in consulting another doctor for a second opinion. It is frequently in confusing these two situations that the patient or the patient's family becomes annoyed and experiences embarrassment or mental anguish. It is wiser however for the patient to know and recognize the situation than to believe that problems do not exist. But by going about it correctly problems can certainly be avoided.

First of all, the important point to remember is that when a person is dissatisfied with his doctor he should simply dismiss him. The doctor should be told politely either in person or by dropping a note to him that his services are no longer required. It is up to the patient whether or not he chooses to tell the doctor why he is leaving him, however I have always thought it a courteous thing to do. In this way a clean break is made. The patient then, if he knows of a different doctor he wishes to consult, can go to him, assured he has done everything possible to alleviate any misunderstanding.

One area where much confusion occurs, unfortunately, is when a patient, in an effort to be courteous to his doctor, phrases his request in such a manner that his doctor, let us say Dr. Smith, offers to call in Dr. Jones as a consultant. Unaware of the problems this may create later, the patient agrees. Upon seeing Dr. Jones he is much impressed with his diagnosis and treatment and feels that Dr. Jones was more thorough and possibly showed more sympathy and understanding of the case than did Dr. Smith.

When the patient wants to go to a doctor again he may want to see Dr. Jones but may be puzzled and annoyed that Dr. Jones says he cannot see him. This is because he is actually Dr. Smith's patient and Dr. Jones was called in only as a consultant. This situation is not infrequent, particularly in smaller communities where there are only a small number of physicians practicing, and of course, the smaller the community the more important it is for people in medicine to work well together.

The important thing for patients to know if they wish to change physicians is that they should not have the doctor to whom they wish to go called in as a consultant. Where human beings are concerned, emotions, hurt feelings and even anger will be present when such circumstances are clumsily handled.

Sometimes, when a patient wants a second medical opinion, he will go to another doctor without telling him he already has a physician. If the diagnosis and treatment are in agreement he may go back to his original doctor satisfied with the care he is receiving.

In most instances a competent and able man will have no

objection to his patient going to another doctor and often will telephone the doctor who has been consulted to tell him so. Or the doctor being consulted, if he is made aware of the circumstances, may feel an obligation to the original doctor to tell him he is seeing his patient and the response will most likely be cordial and understanding.

I was quite amused one day when I dropped in on a former and very able professor of mine, a famous consultant who saw patients only at limited times. I found no less than three of my regular but worrisome patients sitting in his waiting room. Each was greatly embarrassed and in turn went to great lengths to explain to me that they were only taking an extra precaution, concerned that something might have been missed and went on and on. They were greatly relieved when I told them it certainly sounded like a good idea to me! In each case it only served to strengthen our relationship.

Fortunately today, people are learning much more about their own bodies, their own health, and therefore the doctor is not set up as some righteous diety who, alone and without question, understands the intricate and mystical functions and malfunctions of the body. Also the fact that doctors have specialized has eased the situation and patients can move freely and often go to different doctors as they need different services. The previous, awkward situation of changing doctors is one which we most likely inherited from England. There, in the old days, the patient was to a certain degree the property of his doctor. This was true even to the extent that when a doctor retired or moved to a different city he could actually "sell" his practice, and what is even more amazing, in fact deliver it. But today things are changing. If something is not clearing up as it should the family physician who is devoted to his profession and to his patient, will suggest, "Why don't you go see Dr. Jones, he specializes in such problems!"

This is the ideal situation of course, and everyone should be encouraged to seek out and find a doctor on whom they can depend and in whom they can confide; a doctor who will treat them if he feels confident to do so, or who will suggest a specialist and direct them to the best man in the field if he feels the patient's interests would be better served by doing that. In this way doctors can work together *and* individually.

There will be a good exchange of information, including medical records, x-rays and lab tests and this is to the benefit of both the health and the well-being of the patient. Establishing a sound relationship with your doctor is a source of peace of mind in knowing there is someone who has a knowledge of your past medical record to call upon in the event of an emergency; a familiar and dependable *friend* rather than a stranger.

YOUR DOCTOR'S STAFF

Some people tend to expect the doctor himself to handle every aspect of their relationship with his office. When you visit the office you will quickly come into contact with the staff which he has carefully selected to represent him in matters which he feels can be more efficiently handled by them. His concern and attention must be directed toward the care of his patients.

The doctor's office may include simply himself and a receptionist or a nurse. Or, your doctor may employ a receptionist, several nurses, assistants, technicians and a bookkeeper. It is wise to learn the names of these members of his staff and to cooperate with them in all matters which they can handle. By the doctor's direction, they will be the first to tell you if your question is one for which the doctor himself should be consulted.

In order to provide patients with the best possible care and finest medical equipment, often several doctors will form a medical group or conduct their practices from a medical clinic. This is frequently more economical as far as overhead is concerned, plus they have the added advantage of the mutual services of other staff such as bookkeepers, receptionists, technicians and they may even have access to x-ray equipment and test laboratories on the premises. Frequently, these medical groups include a number of specialists and your doctor may wish to call upon one or more of them or refer you to one for a particular problem.

Your financial relationship with your doctor

People pay the milkman, they know what to expect and what their responsibility is when they take the family automobile into a garage for repairs, but frequently they do not take a realistic attitude toward their doctor bills. One of the reasons for this may well be that most doctors have gone to great lengths to provide health care in any event and to avoid causing a financial hardship for their patients.

However, it is incorrect to assume all doctors are rich. The cost of their education is extremely high and it is not unusual for a doctor to be paying off those expenses long after he has graduated from medical school. If he is building a practice, purchasing equipment or getting established in a new area, he may in fact have a problem making ends meet. Additionally, today's soaring costs in general, and the insurance he must carry in particular, can create a tremendously heavy financial burden on him.

You will do yourself and your doctor a favor by discussing his fees and your insurance coverage with his bookkeeper or secretary and learning exactly what you may reasonably expect the insurance to cover and what you will personally be responsible for. Knowing in advance is far preferable to the unpleasant surprise when you *assume* your insurance company will pay for an expensive medical procedure only to learn later that it has been dissallowed. You will generally find your doctor's bookkeeper or other staff member charged with these responsibilities to be helpful, cooperative and often sympathetic. They are experienced in dealing with lengthy and difficult-to-understand forms, and they can be of great assistance to you.

Remember. . .

Finding a better-than-average physician is important to your good health.

Sources for locating such a doctor include:

- recommendation from a previous long-time and trusted physician
- medical directories available at library reference desks
- local medical societies
- national health organizations
- medical schools in your area
- a large and efficient hospital near your home
- a casualty insurance company
- personal recommendation from someone whose judgment you respect
- ideally, a combination of the above

Inquire about your doctor's standard policies and procedures, particularly for emergency care.

If you wish to change doctors, politely tell the one you wish to drop that his services are no longer required. Do not have your doctor call another in as a consultant if what you really want is to change doctors.

Get to know your doctor's staff; go to *them* with questions which fall into *their areas of responsibility.*

Do not hesitate to discuss with your doctor or his staff fees for medical procedures and your insurance coverage.

Chapter Nine

Emergency!

Do you know what to do in the event of an emergency? It may be too late to start finding out after the emergency has occurred and you are the only one around to take charge. There are many very fine books available which go into great detail about the specific actions that should be taken in each situation and it is wise to always have at least one such reference book available.

Additionally, at least one member of a family should have some training in emergency first aid. Classes are given regularly and inexpensively in almost every community through the facilities of YMCA's, community recreation centers or other service-oriented community organizations. Through such classes you learn through actual demonstration by trained professionals and usually will also have the opportunity to practice administering first aid to fellow students in mock emergency settings. Such training is much more effective than is simply reading instructions. In fact, I would encourage family members to take such a course together since it will provide them with vital knowledge as well as a meaningful family experience.

In an emergency, once you have done what is absolutely imperative, such as for example, stopped the bleeding from a severed artery, the most important service you can render to a victim is to get him as quickly as possible into the hands of competent medical professionals.

If you have not acquainted yourself with the emergency facilities available in your community, do so at the first possible opportunity. They vary from state to state and city to city. The first place to turn for this information is the inside front cover of your telephone directory. It is wise to post emergency numbers near the telephone. In many heavily populated communities one call to the Fire Department will bring a rescue unit speeding to your home or scene of the accident or medical emergency. Usually these people are radio-equipped and prepared to transport or arrange for prompt transportation of the victim to the nearest hospital. Often they are backed up by first aid units and more and more commonly by paramedic teams who are in radio contact with the medical staff of a hospital. They can direct ambulances and if there are traffic problems will radio for police escort. They are trained to deal with all phases of emergency service including cardiac arrest. Their efficient handling saves lives daily, but the effectiveness can be greatly aided by the minutes and even seconds gained by prompt notification.

In Chapter Ten I refer to the American College of Emergency Physicians. This group which began in 1961 with four physicians, now has a membership of more than 7,000 who must meet the continuing medical education requirement of 150 hours every three years. Included in their comprehensive effort toward providing the best possible emergency care is a program to coordinate emergency services within the community.

A telephone call to your local fire department with specific questions in mind will give you the information which may save a life, so do find out the proper number to call in your area: DO IT NOW AND KEEP IT CLOSE AT HAND.

Whether or not there is a charge for emergency service varies from one community to another. For example, where emergency services are handled by the local fire department which is funded by taxes, there will probably be no charge. In other areas where there are volunteer fire departments or other plans for handling such problems, there may or may not be a charge. It is best to familiarize yourself in advance with the organization and their policies.

Naturally, the first concern is for the patient or victim. If his life depends on getting treatment immediately, he should be taken to the nearest facility. However, if there is time and if it is possible to obtain the information, he should be taken to the hospital of his choice, preferably to the one where his doctor practices.

Do you know the most direct route to your hospital and on which street the emergency entrance is located? Don't wait until a member of your family is in critical need of medical attention to learn these important facts. Make it your business to drive, and find out how to direct someone else to drive, directly to the emergency entrance. If you are leaving to take someone to a hospital emergency room, ask someone else to call to let them know you are on your way. This is particularly important should you need help in getting the patient from the car into the building. In many instances TIME IS THE MOST IMPORTANT FACTOR. One must be capable of making the decision of whether to call for professional aid or to transport the patient himself. In choosing the latter, precious minutes can be lost by having to look for street names in an unfamiliar area or in driving around a hospital to find a sign directing you to the emergency entrance.

Another situation which presents itself from time to time is when someone becomes ill or falls victim to an accident in a strange city they are visiting. There have been instances when patients have called me long distance to ask where to turn for medical care. If a person gets sick in a hotel, he can, of course, call the hotel physician and ask him to call a specialist, but this does not necessarily lead to securing the best care. Probably the most expedient and the best medical help can be obtained in such a situation by locating a large and efficient hospital and by seeking help through their staff.

Travel always presents a few circumstances which must be taken into consideration. Another problem of which we hear from time to time is when a child either becomes acutely ill or is injured in an accident at a time when his/her parents or guardians are traveling and cannot be reached immediately. Doctors and hospitals must have authorization from the parent or legal guardian of a minor before performing medical or surgical procedures. Time is lost if it becomes necessary to obtain alternative legal authorization in the absence of the parents.

However, it is a relatively uncomplicated matter for parents to write a simply-worded authorization directed to the doctor and hospital to be left with the person in charge of the child while they are gone. Some school districts provide such a form for parents to sign which are kept in the school offices so authorization can be immediately obtained if the child is hurt at school and the parents cannot be reached. It may be hand written and say for example:

____
(date)

Please accept this as our authorization for our family doctor,

______________________________, any doctor available in his

absence and/or the staff of any hospital or medical facility to render whatever medical aid or surgical procedure they

feel is necessary to our child/children ____________________

____

______________________ (signed)   ______________________ (signed)

Be sure it is dated and signed and in the hands of the person with whom the child or children are staying. A small amount of advance planning and precaution can save much worry and avoid possible anguish.

Remember...

Find out what medical emergency services are available in your community before an emergency arises.

Keep emergency information close at hand and see to it that you or a member of your family has training in emergency first aid.

Make a test run to the emergency entrance of your hospital so you will be prepared in the event of an actual crisis.

If you become sick or injured in another city, go to a large hospital for help.

As parents or guardians of minors, be sure to leave your written authorization for medical care in your absence.

Chapter Ten

Specialists

If your regular doctor is a family practitioner it is quite possible that he will suggest the services of a specialist from time to time. For example, a family physician may send a patient to a surgeon for consultation if there is a question of whether or not surgery is necessary, and if it is, to perform the surgery. Generally when a specialist in a certain field is required, your doctor will ask if you have someone in mind and if you do not, he will give you a choice of several capable doctors in that field.

Following is a list of specialists and a brief description of the field of medicine and treatment for which they have taken extensive study and acquired experience. An asterisk (*) indicates specialties recognized by the American Medical Association. Each requires four years of medical school an M.D. degree, plus two to six additional years of residency training in the specialty.

*ANESTHESIOLOGIST—a physician specializing in anesthesiology (causing the patient to be insensitive to touch, pain or other stimulation) in distinction to an anesthetist who may or may not be a physician.

*ALLERGIST—a physician who specializes in the hypersensitivity of the body cells to a specific substance resulting in various reactions. This branch of medicine embraces the study, diagnosis and treatment of allergic manifestation.

ANESTHETIST—one who produces anesthesia by administration of an anesthetic.

*CARDIOLOGIST—a physician having special knowledge of and experience in the diagnosis and treatment of heart disease.

CHIROPODIST/PODIATRIST—a practitioner who treats diseases, injuries and defects of the human foot.

*DERMATOLOGIST—a physician who specializes in the diagnosis and treatment of diseases of the skin; a skin specialist.

ENDOCRINOLOGIST—a specialist in the science dealing with the glands of internal secretion and their function and activities, disorders or disease.

*FAMILY PHYSICIAN/GENERAL PRACTITIONER—a physician trained to take care of the majority of non-surgical diseases, sometimes including obstetrics.

*GASTROENTEROLOGIST—a physician who specializes in diseases of the stomach and intestine.

*GERATRIC PHYSICIAN—one specializing in the science of old age; dealing with the function and activities, disorders and disease of organs, tissues and cells of the elderly.

*GYNECOLOGIST—a physician in the branch of medicine having to do with diseases of women, primarily those of the genital tract as well as female endocrinology and reproductive functions.

*INTERNIST—a physician trained in internal medicine for adults and specializing in diagnosis and treatment as distinguished from a surgeon, obstetrician or other specialist.

*NEUROLOGIST—a physician specializing in the treatment of

nervous diseases and the branch of medical science that has to do with the nervous system and its disorders.

*OBSTETRICIAN—a physician skilled in the medical care of women during pregnancy and childbirth.

*OPTHAMOLOGIST—a physician who is a specialist in the anatomy, physiology and diseases and refractive errors of the eye; may perform surgery, prescribe medicine, and optical aids such as corrective lenses.

OPTICIAN—one who makes and adjusts eyeglasses and spectacles from a prescription supplied by an opthamologist or optometrist.

OPTOMETRIST—a person trained and licensed to examine and test the eyes and to treat visual defects by prescribing and adapting corrective lenses and other optical aids and establishing programs of exercises.

*ORTHOPEDIST—a physician who deals with the skeletal system; a specialist who is concerned with the preservation, restoration and development of the bones and joints by medical, surgical and physical methods.

*OSTEOPATH—a physician with at least four years of medical training with emphasis on manipulative techniques of the skeletal system supported by the use of medicines, surgery, proper diet and other therapy.

*OTOLARYNGOLOGIST—a physician who deals with the combined specialties of diseases of the ear and larynx, often including the upper respiratory tract and many diseases of the head and neck, trachea, bronchial tract and esophagus.

*PATHOLOGIST—a doctor of medicine who practices chiefly in the laboratory serving as a consultant to his clinical colleagues (especially with reference to diagnosis of tissue removed for biopsy and selection of diagnostic tests and interpretation of laboratory results.)

*PEDIATRICIAN—a physician who specializes in the treatment of children.

PHARMACIST—a druggist, one who prepares and dispenses

drugs and has knowledge concerning their properties.

PHARMACOLOGIST—one who specializes in the science that deals with drugs, their sources, appearance, chemistry, actions and uses.

*PSYCHIATRIST—a physician who specializes in the diagnosis and treatment of mental disease.

PSYCHOLOGIST—one who deals with the science of the mind and behavior.

*PULMONARY SPECIALIST—a physician specializing in the medical treatment of disorders relating to the lungs.

*RADIOLOGIST—a physician skilled in the diagnostic and therapeutic use of x-rays and forms of radiant energy.

*SURGEON—a physician who performs operations or treats accidents or diseases responsive to operative or manual treatment.

*THORACTIC SURGEON—a physician dealing in the diagnosis and surgical treatment of disorders pertaining to the chest, heart and lungs.

*UROLOGIST—a physician who specializes in the study, diagnosis and treatment of the genitourinary tract (organs concerned with the functions of reproduction and urination).

As one can see simply by reading the above, many of the medical specialties overlap and the descriptions given here are extremely brief and limited due to space.

Chapter Eleven

Community Services

Many people would be pleasantly surprised if they would take the initiative to learn more about the community services provided in their vicinity. This is particularly true in metropolitan areas although even rural areas usually have facilities available in the nearest town or county seat, and in many instances even transportation is provided if that is a problem. Often there are visiting nurse services available, too.

Services provided cover a broad range and typical organizations will include such things as a family health clinic which is concerned with family planning (often in conjunction with Planned Parenthood); child health care for the purpose of keeping well children well through physical examinations, immunizations, parental counseling; tests for tuberculosis and sickle cell anemia; physical examinations for senior citizens; nutrition information and a myriad of other services.

By calling the Department of Public Health and Welfare listed under the name of the county in which you live, information can be given by phone or mailed to you. For example, in the area of developmentally disabled children and adults which may cover autism, cerebral palsy, epilepsy, mental retardation and other neurologically handicapping conditions, doctors and medical aid including diagnosis and counseling are often provided. Further, one can obtain information concerning schools, recreation for handicapped children and adults, financial aid, out-of-town care and even job information. Another influential resource is the parent or family group which joins together and provides an opportunity to talk over problems, compare experiences and do much to help both the patient and his/her family.

I want to stress here that it is important that you not become discouraged if your initial effort or first contact does not result in the help you need. You must be persistent in your efforts to find the agencies and services that will be the most valuable to you. Depending upon the organization, some services are provided without charge, others have fees which are based on income. These are, however, organizations which were designed to provide the best possible help available and one should not hesitate to make use of the services they provide. No amount of money can buy the fine professional help and emotional support offered.

Visiting Nurses Associations are a source of hope and health by providing care to the sick in the home including teaching family members to care for the patient or the patient how to care for himself. Sometimes there is also a homemaker/home-health-aide program which will provide such services as sponge baths and showers; help with cane, crutches and walkers; prescribed exercises; child care; light housekeeping; laundry; meal planning, preparation and serving; assisting with doctor appointments, shopping and doing errands and in general providing emotional and physical support. Additionally they may be able to provide a nurse, physical therapist, occupational therapist and/or speech therapists within the community and, in many instances, in the home.

Probably the greatest strides in providing information and help have been in the area of mental health. There are education and consultation services including communication skills courses for the entire family when one feels their home suffers from a lack of cooperation, a lack of respect for other family members' feelings, or simply needs a more open exchange of ideas. There are day centers and continuing care programs, outpatient services which include short-term counseling and treatment, in-patient services and crisis intervention services.

The quality and number of services available vary greatly from community to community and often, because they are listed under different names in different localities, the biggest problem is in locating them. Most likely, your doctor or a member of his staff can get you started in the right direction. Also, check carefully your telephone directory or the directory of the largest city near your home under such listings as Health Organizations, Public Health, listings under the name of the state, county and city Health Services, Health and Welfare Department, or alphabetically for Cancer Society, Crippled Children Society, Diabetes Association, etc. However, a call first either to the County Medical Society or to the Department of Health and Welfare will probably provide the correct names of the organizations and probably the local telephone numbers which you seek. They can also give you information on whom to call for medical emergencies, suicide prevention, poison information, occupational health services for work-related health problems, rodent and insect control, drug abuse information, etc.

It is good to know where to turn for help. I have one friend and patient who will be forever grateful to a member of my staff who provided her with the telephone number which brought prompt help when a swarm of bees entered her open window to set up what threatened to be a health hazard in her bedroom. As she watched from the neighbor's window, a state-commissioned beekeeper carried the queen bee out of her home followed by the swarm. Soon order was restored, the woman reclaimed her bedroom, and the bees were taken to a more appropriate residence.

There are community services to help you cope with sudden, short-term incidents as well as with permanently disabling illnesses. But remember, large or small, your problem probably is not unique. We are fortunate that through the experience and efforts of others who have had to learn to cope and to live with similar problems, illnesses and disabilities, there are now places to turn to for help, and more than likely there are facilities close to home.

Remember. . .

Community services were designed to help you, but you must make your needs known. Be persistent in looking for the agencies and services available.

These services have access to the finest professionals in their field and can provide physical and emotional support that is not available elsewhere at any price.

Chapter Twelve

Health Organizations

On a much larger scale there are national and even international organizations which are administered by and whose members include the top echelon of medical men in their field. These organizations, societies, associations, foundations, programs and institutes were usually formed to promote professional research and study, to exchange current theories and methods of treatment, to raise funds to combat the disease, and to provide training grants for research and study.

In this chapter I am listing the national offices of what I feel is a comprehensive number providing the widest range of information on various problems. Many of these national organizations have local offices. However, when one does not know how to go about obtaining a source of information, I would suggest contacting the national headquarters. They, most likely, can assist you in finding appropriate medical help in your vicinity. Many have a special committee in the national organization whose responsibility it is to provide information to individuals. In fact, some of these organizations provide such extensive services that space has not permitted even a partial listing here. Where it is indicated that they provide information and educational materials to the public, it may be worthwhile to explain your particular needs when writing to them. In addition to the informational materials, they will probably also refer you to their affiliated office nearest your home. You might also ask for the names of other organizations concerned with your particular problem. For example, there are probably six or eight national organizations concerned with the blind, but space limitations have precluded a complete listing here.

AGING—Gerontological Society, One Dupont Circle, Suite 520, Washington D.C., 20036—Publishes information about aging for anyone interested in improving the health and well-being of older people and bringing together all groups interested in their care.

ALLERGY—Allergy Foundation of America, 801 Second Avenue, New York, New York, 10017—Concerned with hay fever, asthma, skin disorders, allergic reactions to drugs, foods and insect stings. Provides information and educational materials to the public.

ARTHRITIS—Arthritis Foundation, 1212 Avenue of the Americas, New York, New York, 10036—Extends knowledge of arthritis and other rheumatic diseases to the lay public emphasizing socioeconomic as well as medical aspects of these diseases.

BIRTH—American Association for Maternal and Child Care, P. O. Box 965, Los Altos, California, 94022—Publishes *American Baby* for mothers-to-be as well as reprints concerning prenatal and postnatal care.

Rubella Birth Defect Evaluation Project, c/o Roosevelt Hospital, 428 West 59th Street, New York, New York, 10019. Information and educational materials.

BLIND—National Society for the Prevention of Blindness, 79 Madison Avenue, New York, New York, 10016—Conducts nationwide comprehensive programs for public and professional education, research and industrial and community services.

American Foundation for the Blind, 15 West 16th Street, New York, New York, 10011—Conducts public education programs. Publishes *New Outlook for the Blind* and a directory of agencies serving the visually handicapped. Develops and manufactures special aids for blind persons.

BLOOD—American Association of Blood Banks, 1828 L Street, N.W., Washington, D.C. 20036—Provides information concerning blood banks.

National Hemophilia Foundation, 25 West 39th Street, New York, New York, 10018—Disseminates literature to the general public, offers referral services for patients, sponsors summer camps for young hemophiliacs.

Association for Sickle Cell Anemia, 520 Fifth Avenue, New York, New York, 10036—conducts educational programs to inform the public about sickle cell anemia and assists families of persons with sickle cell anemia. Pamphlet available.

BRAIN—Brain Research Foundation, University of Chicago, 343 South Dearborn Street, Chicago, Illinois, 60604—Fosters clinical and related professional care for persons afflicted with brain disease.

BURN—International Society for Burn Injuries, 4200 East Ninth Avenue. C-309, Denver, Colorado, 80220—Seeks to disseminate knowledge and stimulate prevention in the field of burns; promotes and coordinates scientific, clinical and social research on burn education in all phases of burn care.

CANCER—American Cancer Society, 219 East 42nd Street, New York, New York, 10017—Publishes brochures and provides information and educational materials to the public; provides special services for cancer patients.

CEREBRAL PALSY—United Cerebral Palsy Associations, 66 East 34th Street, New York, New York, 10016—Supports and provides information regarding local affiliates; provides treatment, therapy, vocational training, recreational facilities for children and adults, home instruction, psychological guidance for parents. Provides services in areas not served by local affiliates.

CHEST—Research and Education Foundation for Chest Disease, 911 Busse Highway, Park Ridge, Illinois, 60068—Provides information and educational materials.

CHILDREN—National Society for Autistic Children, 169 Tampa Avenue, Albany, New York, 12208—Provides information to the public of the symptoms and problems of the autistic child to promote a better understanding of the condition. National information and referral services.

Foundation for Child Development, 345 East 46th Street, New York, New York, 10017—Formerly the Association for the Aid of Crippled Children. Provides information and educational materials to the public.

CYSTIC FIBROSIS—Cystic Fibrosis Foundation, 3379 Peachtree Road, N.E., Atlanta, Georgia, 30326—Provides information and public health education programs on the most common inherited fatal disease among caucasians; provides care centers and various services for young adults with cystic fibrosis.

DEAF—National Association for the Deaf, 814 Thayer Avenue, Silver Spring, Maryland, 20910—Strives to provide information, prevent discrimination, promote economic, intellectual, professional and social betterment of the deaf.

DENTAL—American Dental Association, 211 East Chicago Avenue, Chicago, Illinois, 60611—Provides information and educational materials to the public.

DIABETES—American Diabetes Association, One West 48th Street, New York, New York, 10020—Publishes *Forecast* (bimonthly) for diabetics and their families; distributes accurate information to the public; develops educational methods to give diabetic patients a better understanding of their disease.

DIGESTION—American Digestive Disease Society, 295 Madison Avenue, New York, New York, 10017—(Gastroenterology)—Strives to educate the public concerning the nature and treatment, as well as the prevention of digestive diseases which affect twenty-two million Americans.

DRUGS—American Pharmaceutical Association, 2215 Constitution Avenue, N.W., Washington, D.C., 20037—Strives to improve and promote public health by aiding in the establishment of satisfactory standards for drugs and to aid in the detection and prevention of adulteration and misbranding of drugs and medicine.

EMERGENCY—American College of Emergency Physicians, 241 East Saginaw, Suite 550, East Lansing, Michigan, 48823—Aim is improving emergency department care in hospitals and coordinating emergency services within the community among those concerned, such as policemen, firemen and ambulance attendants.

ENDOCRINE—Endocrine Society, 9650 Rockville Pike, Bethesda, Maryland, 20014—Provides information and educational materials.

EPILEPSY—Epilepsy Foundation of America, 1828 L Street, N.W., Suite 406, Washington, D.C., 20036—Acts as spokesman and advocate for four million Americans with epilepsy; defines the myriads of problems and devises specific programs to solve them.

EYES—American Association of Opthalmology, 1100 17th Street, N.W., Washington, D.C., 20036—Provides information and educational materials concerning eye care.

FEET—American Podiatry Association, 20 Chevy Chase Circle, N.W., Washington, D.C., 20015—Provides information and educational materials.

First Aid—International Rescue and First Aid Association, 5201 Madison Road, Cincinnati, Ohio, 45227—Provides information and educational materials.

Health—American Public Health Association, 1015 18th Street, N.W., Washington, D.C., 20036—Provides information on all individual health and medical organizations.

American Health Foundation, 1370 Avenue of the Americas, New York, New York, 10019—Promotes preventative medicine and provides educational materials and information.

Heart—American Heart Association, 44 East 23rd Street, New York, New York, 10010—Provides information and educational materials to the public.

Kidney—National Kidney Foundation, 116 East 27th Street, New York, New York, 10016—Provides patient services, professional and public information; Organ Donor Program; community services.

Leukemia—Leukemia Society of America, 211 East 43rd Street, New York, New York, 10017—Provides information and educational materials as well as aid to needy patients; publishes brochures.

Lung—American Lung Association, 1740 Broadway, New York, New York, 10019—Formerly the National Tuberculosis and Respiratory Disease Association. Provides information and educational materials.

Mental Health—American Association for Mental Deficiency, 5201 Connecticut, N.W., Washington, D.C., 20015—Provides information and educational materials.

National Association for Mental Health, 1800 North Kent Street, Rosslyn, Virginia, 22209—Provides information and educational materials.

Institute for Bioenergetic Analysis, 144 East 36th Street, No. 1A, New York, New York, 10016—Provides information on mental and physical health as related to biological energy processes.

MULTIPLE SCLEROSIS—National Multiple Sclerosis Society, 257 Park Avenue South, New York, New York, 10010—Provides services and aid for disabled patients and their families including those with multiple sclerosis and related disorders of the central nervous system.

MUSCULAR DYSTROPHY—Muscular Dystrophy Associations of America, 810 Seventh Avenue, New York, New York, 10019—Publishes general and technical literature; renders services to patients locally through affiliated chapters; provides orthopedic appliances, therapy, flu shots and conducts summer camps for those afflicted with muscular dystrophy.

NERVES—National Committee for Research in Neurological Disorders, 927 Park Avenue South, New York, New York, 10010—Provides information and educational materials concerning nervous disorders.

NURSING—National Federation of Licensed Practical Nurses, 250 West 57th Street, New York, New York, 10019—Provides information concerning nursing care.

American Health Care Association, 1200 15th Street, N.W., Washington, D.C., 20005—Provides information and educational materials regarding nursing home care.

NUTRITION—American Dietetic Association, 430 North Michigan Avenue, Chicago, Illinois, 60611—Provides information and educational materials on diet and nutrition.

ORTHOPEDIC—American Orthopaedic Association, 430 North Michigan Avenue, Chicago, Illinois, 60611— Provides information to further knowledge in diagnosis and treatment of crippling diseases.

PATHOLOGY—Intersociety Committee on Pathology Information (Information Services, Inc.) 9650 Rockville Pike, Bethesda, Maryland, 20014.

PARAPLEGIA—National Paraplegia Foundation, 333 North

Michigan Avenue, Chicago, Illinois, 60601—Strives to inform and educate the public and to participate actively in the rehabilitation and community services available to individuals.

PHYSICAL THERAPY—American Physical Therapy Association, 1156 15th Street, N.W., Washington, D.C., 20005—Provides informational materials.

American Academy of Physical Medicine and Rehabilitation, 30 North Michigan Avenue, Chicago, Illinois, 60602—Promotes use of physical therapy and rehabilitation in treatment of arthritics, poliomyelitis victims, cerebral palsey victims, amputees, etc.

PSORIASIS—Psoriasis Research Association, 107 Vista Del Grande, San Carlos, California, 94070.—Provides information and educational materials.

PSYCHIATRY—American Psychiatric Association, 1700 18th Street, N.W., Washington, D.C., 20009—Provides information and educational materials.

SKIN—American Academy of Dermatology 116 South Fifth, Tacoma, Washington, 98405—Provides information and educational materials concerning the skin and skin diseases and disorders.

SURGERY—American College of Surgeons, 55 East Erie Street, Chicago, Illinois, 60611—Provides informational and reference materials.

VENEREAL DISEASE—American Venereal Disease Association, 401 College Avenue, Norfolk, Virginia, 23507—Conducts public service programs and provides informational material for the diagnosis, treatment and control of venereal disease.

Remember. . .

The organizations listed here represent only a partial number, and in most cases their primary goal is toward research and study of a particular disease or problem.

As a service to the public, most of them will provide information to individuals, particularly where to go for assistance in your community.

Many provide extensive services to patients and their families. Their help may be invaluable to you.

BIBLIOGRAPHY

Alfred, J. Tyrone and Cannon, Alfred C. *Medical Handbook For The Layman.* Port Washington, N.Y.: Alfred, 1969

American National Red Cross. *Advanced First Aid And Emergency Care.* New York: Doubleday & Co., 1973.

Andreopoulos, Spyros. *Primary Care: Where Medicine Fails.* New York: John Wiley & Sons, 1975.

Arnold, Robert E. *What To Do About Bites & Stings Of Venomous Animals.* New York: Macmillan, 1973.

Augenstein, Leroy G. *Come, Let Us Play God.* New York: Harper & Row, 1969.

Better Homes & Gardens/Editors. *Better Homes & Gardens Family Medical Guide.* Des Moines, Iowa: Meredith Corp., 1973.

Bredow, Miriam. *Handbook For The Medical Secretary.* New York: McGraw-Hill, 1963.

Brown, Warren J. *Patients' Guide To Medicine.* Fallbrook, Ca.,: Aero Medical, 1973.

Burdock, Eugene I. and Hardesty, Anne S. *Structured Clinical Interview.* New York: Springer Publishing Company, 1969.

Carter, James P., et al. *Keeping Your Family Healthy Overseas.* New York: Seymour Lawrence, 1971.

Chatton, Milton J. *Handbook of Medical Treatment.* Los Altos, Ca.: Lange, 1974.

Chisari, Francis V., M.D., and Nakamura, Robert. *Consumer's Guide to Health Care.* Boston: Little, Brown and Company, 1976.

Clark, Duncan W., and MacMahon, Brian W. *Preventive Medicine.* Boston: Little, Brown and Company, 1967.

Clark, Randolph L., and Cumley, Russell W. *The Book of Health,* 3rd edition. New York: Van Nostrand, Reinhold, 1973.

Coe, Rodney M., and Brehm, Henry P. *Preventive Health Care for Adults.* New Haven, Conn.: College & University Press, 1972.

Current Medical Information And Terminology, 4th edition. Chicago: AMA, 1971.

Del Guercio, Louis R. *Multilingual Manual For Medical History-Taking.* Boston: Little, Brown, 1972.

DiCyan, Erwin, and Hessman, Lawrence. *Without Prescription.* New York: Simon & Schuster, 1972.

Directory of Medical Specialists, 2 Vols., 17th edition. Chicago: Marquis, 1975.

Doyle, Patrick J. *Save Your Health And Your Money.* Washington, D.C.: Acropolis Books, 1971.

Edwards, Marvin H. *Hazardous To Your Health.* New York: Arlington House, 1972.

Enelow, Allen J., and Swisher, Scott. *Interviewing And Patient Care.* New York: Oxford University Press, 1972.

Ferguson, L. Kraeer, and Kerr, John H. *Explain It To Me, Doctor.* Philadelphia: J. B. Lippincott Company, 1971.

Findeiss, J. Clifford. *Emergency Medical Care.* New York: Stratton Intercon, 1974.

Fishbein, Morris, M.D. *Popular Medical Encyclopedia.* New York: Doubleday & Company, Inc., 1946.

Gaver, Jessyca R. *Complete Directory of Medical & Health Services.* New York: Award Books, 1970.

Greco, Ray S., and Pittenger, Rex A. *One Man's Practice: Effects Of Developing Insight On Doctor-Patient Transactions.* Philadelphia: J. B. Lippincott, 1966.

Greenblatt, Augusta. *Questions Young People Ask About Their Health.* New York: Pyramid, 1974.

Hicks, Dorothy J. *Patient Care Techniques.* New York: Bobbs-Merrill, 1975.

Hudson, Ian, and Thomas, Gordon. *What To Do Until The Doctor Comes.* New York: Mason/Charter Publishers, Inc., 1969.

Hurdle, J. Frank. *A Country Doctor's Common Sense Health Manual.* Englewood Cliffs, N.J.: Prentice-Hall, 1975.

Jaco, E. Gartly. *Patients, Physicians and Illness.* New York: Free Press, 1972.

Johnson, G. Timothy. *Doctor: What You Should Know About Health Care Before You Call A Physician.* New York: McGraw- Hill Book Company, 1975.

Kennedy, Edward F. *In Critical Condition.* New York: Simon & Schuster, 1973.

Kime, Robert E. *Health: A Consumer's Dilemma.* Palo Alto: Wadsworth Publishing Co., 1970.

Kinney, C., et al. *Doctor's Quick Guide To Home Treatments For Over 200 Common Ailments.* Englewood Cliffs, N.J.: Parker Publishing Company, 1972.

Kordel, Lelord. *You're Younger Than You Think: The Mature Person's Guide to Vibrant Health.* New York: G. P. Putnam's Sons, 1976.

Levin, Arthur L. *Talk Back To Your Doctor: How to Demand (and Recognize) High Quality Health Care.* New York: Doubleday & Co., 1975.

Levy, Joseph V., and Bach-y-Rita, Paul. *Vitamins: Their Use And Abuse.* New York: Liveright, 1976.

Lipkin, Mack. *Care Of Patients: Concepts And Tactics.* New York: Oxford University Press, 1974.

Miller, Benjamin F., and Galton, Lawrence. *Family Book Of Preventive Medicine.* New York: Simon & Schuster, 1971.

Miller, Henry, and Hall, Reginald. *Modern Medical Treatment.* Philadelphia: J. B. Lippincott, 1975.

Nourse, Alan E. *The Ladies' Home Journal Family Medical Guide.* New York: Harper & Row, 1973.

Osgood, David, and Copans, Stu. *The Home Health Handbook.* Brattleboro, Vt.: Stephen Greene Press, 1972.

Patrick, Fisher J. *Basic Medical Terminology.* New York: Bobbs-Merrill, 1975.

Pfeiffer, Carl C. *Mental And Elementary Nutrients: A Physician's Guide to Health Care.* New Canaan, Conn.: Keats

Publishing Co., 1975.

Placere, Morris N., and Warwick, Charles A. *How You Can Get Better Medical Care For Less Money.* New York: Walker & Co., 1973.

Prichard, Robert W., and Robinson, Robert E. *Twenty Thousand Medical Words.* New York: McGraw-Hill, 1972.

Reynolds, Frank W., and Barsam, P. C. *Adult Health: Services For The Chronically Ill and Aged.* New York: Macmillan, 1967.

Rothenberg, Robert E. *The New Illustrated Medical Encyclopedia For Home Use,* 4 volumes. New York: Harry N. Abrams, Inc., 1959.

Rutstein, David A. *A Blueprint For Medical Care.* Boston: MIT Press, 1974.

Schifferes, Justus J. *Schifferes Family Medical Encyclopedia.* New York: Pocket Books, 1959.

Schmidt, Alice M., R.N. *The Homemaker's Guide to Home Nursing.* Salt Lake City: Brigham Young University Press, 1976.

Schwartz, Harry. *The Case For American Medicine.* New York: David McKay, 1973.

Snapper, Isadore, and Kahn, Alvin I. *Bedside Medicine.* Philadelphia: Grune & Stratton, 1967.

Taylor, Robert B. *Common Problems In Office Practice.* New York: Harper & Row, 1972.

Wechsler, Henry. *Handbook of Medical Specialties.* New York: Human Sciences Press, 1976.

Willeford, George. *Medical Word Finder.* Englewood Cliffs, N.J.: Prentice-Hall, 1967.